KINESIOLOGY
TAPING
for Rehab and
Injury Prevention

KINESIOLOGY TAPING

for Rehab and Injury Prevention

An Easy, At-Home Guide for Overcoming
Common Strains, Pains and Conditions

Aliana Kim

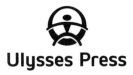

Ulysses Press

Published in the United States by
Ulysses Press
P.O. Box 3440
Berkeley, CA 94703
www.ulyssespress.com

ISBN13: 978-1-61243-553-4
Library of Congress Control Number 2015952127

Printed in the United States by Bang Printing
10 9 8 7 6 5 4 3 2 1

Acquisitions editor: Casie Vogel
Managing editor: Claire Chun
Editor: Lily Chou
Proofreader: Renee Rutledge
Cover design: what!design @ whatweb.com
Interior design: Jake Flaherty
Interior images: Rapt Productions except from shutterstock.com page 13 © f9photos (supine/prone); page 13 © Blamb (planes); page 14 © Mihai Blanaru; page 15 © Mihai Blanaru (adduction/rotation), © Artem Furman (supination), © Pikoso.kz (pronation), © LeventeGyori (dorsiflexion); page 17 © stihii; page 18 © Peter Hermes Furian
Cover images: © Rapt Productions except rolls of tape © nito/shutterstock.com; man in anatomical position © Cliparea | Custom Media/shutterstock.com
Models: Nadia Qabazard, Michael Toy
Index: Sayre Van Young

Distributed by Publishers Group West

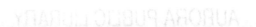

To my husband, who has been my biggest supporter.
Also, to my clients, who have taught me so much about
real-life application over the years that this book would not be possible without them.

CONTENTS

WHAT IS KINESIOLOGY TAPING?

Kinesiology taping is used as temporary treatment for acute and subacute conditions. It can be used to aid those with chronic pain conditions such as arthritis, tennis elbow, patellar tracking syndrome, ankle sprains, carpal tunnel, inflammation, general pain, and structural misalignment. Kinesiology taping can also be used to prevent injuries and help return the body to homeostasis in cases of lymphatic damage like inflammation.

BACKGROUND

Kinesiology taping was developed by Dr. Kenzo Kase in 1979. A licensed chiropractor as well as a licensed acupuncturist, Dr. Kase saw that manual therapy was extremely effective for pain management and overall health, but the effects were usually temporary. He developed kinesiology taping in order to increase the effectiveness of manual therapy. Kinesiology taping was introduced in the United States in 1995, and then introduced to Europe in 1996.

The usage of kinesiology taping varies. People who've had surgeries use it in order to regain some structural function and alignment in the body. Athletes use kinesiology taping in order to keep the body in proper alignment; they also treat it as a preventative measure in regard to injuries. Everyday people use kinesiology taping for maintenance, pain, and proper alignment.

It can be difficult to tape yourself so many turn to doctors of physical therapy (DPT), athletic trainers, massage therapists, kinesiologists, chiropractors, sports medicine physicians, physical therapy assistants, and acupuncturists, just to name a few. Kinesiology taping is really meant for everyone, not just elite athletes. It's especially beneficial for those who are going through some sort of rehabilitation due to injury.

The science of kinesiology taping is still ongoing. There have been studies to support kinesiology taping, but there are also studies that suggest it's nothing more than the placebo effect. The sample sizes tend to be fairly small and, until more research is completed about this therapy, the scientific community will be 50/50 on the subject.

In my own personal practice, it has been extremely useful, specifically when used post-manual therapy. Having worked with a variety of clients, including gunshot victims, I've noticed a drastic difference, especially with lymphatic taping in severely inflamed areas. Until more substantial information comes out in regard to kinesiology taping, it really depends on your own personal practice. I highly recommend that all taping techniques follow some sort of manual therapy. In my own experience, I've gotten the best results this way. It can be beneficial to use taping before a competition as a preventative measure, but it really only turns into a Band-Aid if serious injury occurs.

SAFETY

Before taping, it's important to know that it's fairly new and there isn't a lot of research on the subject. Many, however, have felt the benefits of taping when working with other trained professionals. Taping should always be used in conjunction with other rehabilitative care, such as seeing a physical therapist, chiropractor, massage therapist, or athletic trainer.

Kinesiology taping was never supposed to be used alone for any condition. It was created to prolong care during chiropractic treatment plans. So it's safe to say that if you decide to tape yourself (say, for a chronic condition), be sure to work with a professional rehabilitation therapist first.

This work is meant to enhance the work of your therapist, not replace actual hands-on work with your therapist. Doing soft tissue work makes you feel amazing at the moment but sometimes the effects don't last. Kinesiology taping strives to prolong the effects of soft tissue work.

Disclaimer: None of the taping techniques in this book are meant to treat, diagnose, or cure any disease or ailment. They are purely therapeutic and meant only for educational purposes, and it's highly advised that you seek the help of your physician for any conditions in this book or any condition that causes severe pain, inflammation, neuropathy, hematomas, heat to the area, and bruising. It's always advised to speak to your doctor before attempting to tape yourself, and it's important to check for any underlying conditions before taping.

I hope these basic techniques help you get a grasp of what taping is about. I wish you luck on your taping journey and, as always, be careful and speak to your provider if you choose to use kinesiology taping.

CHAPTER 1
BASIC TERMS

In order to perform kinesiology taping on yourself, there are a few terms you need to know. In this chapter, we'll go over basic anatomy and kinesiology terms that will help you on your journey to self-taping.

It's important to know what exactly kinesiology taping is. Kinesiology taping falls under a separate modality in the rehabilitative fields, similar to the Graston Technique. In most cases, in order to be certified in kinesiology taping, an individual must undergo three stages of training and then take a test offered through Kinesio Taping Association International (KTAI). The tape is meant to enhance the physiological systems of the body in regard to superficial tissue. The purpose of the tape is to prolong any manual therapy that a person has received in that the tape can be worn for up to five days. This has since evolved. Now taping has been used to prevent injury by helping the body stay in a structurally safe position during exercise or competition. It can also alleviate pain if an individual is going through competition slightly injured. As you'll see in the next few chapters, with certain issues kinesiology taping can help with inflammation while simultaneously keeping the area stable and controlling some of the pain.

ANATOMICAL TERMS

Think of this as a rough sketch of anatomical terms you'll see throughout this book. Anatomical terms tell us direction in regard to the body. Instead of using words like "left," "right," "up," or "down," these terms are more specific and will make taping easier to learn. You can always check back to this section if you need a refresher during the taping process.

Anatomical position is when the body is standing erect, toes forward, arms by your sides, and palms facing the same direction as the head (forward).

Positions

Supine position refers to a person lying on their back, with the face facing upward. The *prone* position refers to a person lying on their stomach, face facing down.

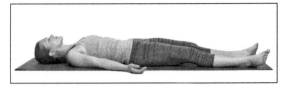

Supine position

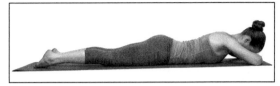

Prone position

Planes of Motion

Some of these have an "alternate" term, but these are the most commonly used. The *sagittal plane* runs vertically and divides the body into left and right halves. The *frontal (coronal) plane* runs vertically and divides the body into front and back portions. The *transverse plane* runs parallel and divides the body into upper and lower portions.

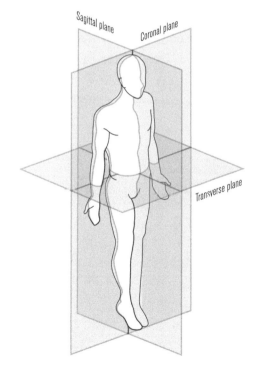

Planes of motion

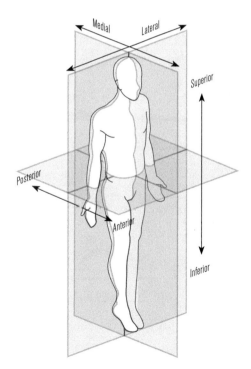

Directions and positions

Directions & Positions

As you use this book as reference, it's important to understand directions and positions when it comes to the body. When you tape, you'll constantly use terms such as adduction, abduction, superior, inferior, and others. These exact terms make it easier for us to identify where tape needs to go. When we say "adduction," we know we want to bring the structure closer to the body. Using proper terms shortens what we have to say in the long run versus saying a mouthful to try to figure out where the structure is in conjunction to what you're trying to tape. Being exact, in any rehabilitative field, is important. We don't want to guess; we want to be 100% sure.

Superior means structures near the head region, usually synonymous with the term "cephalic." *Inferior* is usually synonymous with the word "caudal," which refers to structures near the tail, so think lower body. *Posterior* means back, and *anterior* means front. If you split the body using the frontal plane, this will give you reference to posterior and anterior positions and structures. *Medial* means structures near the midline of the body while *lateral* means structures away from the midline (think appendages). If you split the body by the sagittal plane, this will give you reference to structures that are medial or lateral. Closer to the center cut means the structure is medial. Farther away from the center cut means the structure is more lateral. These two terms are normally in reference to appendages and the axial skeleton.

Movements

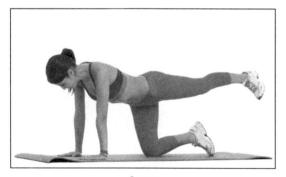

Extension

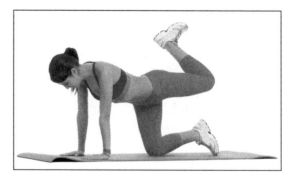

Flexion

These terms are probably the most important and the most used when you start taping. *Extension* straightens or opens a joint. *Flexion* bends a joint or brings bones closer together. *Adduction* brings limbs closer to the midline (think "add"—add to the body). *Abduction* moves limbs away from the midline.

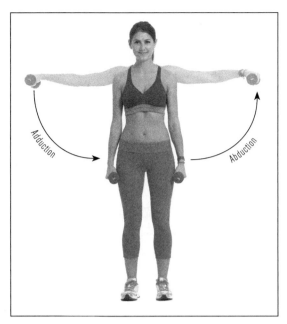

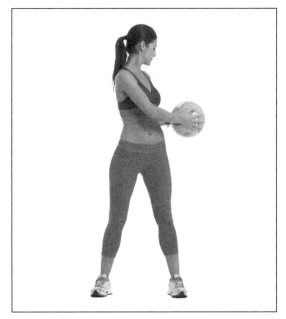

Adduction/Abduction

Rotation

Rotation refers to the axial skeleton and usually happens along the transverse plane. Think of when you look left to right with your head. *Supination* is a pivoting action of the forearm, such as when your palms turn up to hold a bowl of soup. *Pronation* is when the palms face down toward the ground.

Inversion and *eversion* are movements associated with the feet. Inversion pulls the soles of the feet medially. Eversion essentially turns the feet outward and the soles of the feet are lateral. Plantar flexion and dorsiflexion refer to ankle movements. *Plantar flexion* moves the ankle so that the toes push toward the ground. *Dorsiflexion* moves the ankle so that the toes are pulled away from the ground (toes up).

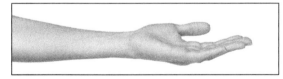

Supination

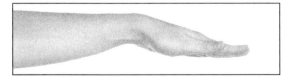

Pronation

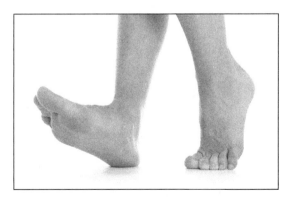

Dorsiflexion (left) and plantar flexion (right).

Muscles

The body has three types of muscle tissue: smooth, cardiac, and skeletal. Smooth muscle is found in our digestive tract while cardiac muscle is found in the heart. Skeletal muscle is connected to our skeletal system and is what makes us move. In this book, we focus solely on skeletal muscle.

When we look at skeletal muscle tissue, it is good to look at it in layers. The epimysium, or outer layer, wraps the entire muscle; it's what incorporates our fascia. (Fascia is a thin, connective sheet; muscular fascia separates individual muscles and muscle groups in the body.) The middle layer, known as the perimysium, covers each bundle of muscle fibers, or fascicle. The deeper layer, called the endomysium, surrounds each individual muscle fiber. Each muscle comes together at the tendon. The tendon attaches the muscle to a bone structure, which gives us the ability to move.

While you are examining the body with your hands during treatment (the palpation process), be aware that when skeletal muscle is not contracted, it has a fairly soft feel, which can make it slightly difficult to find certain landmarks. If you contract the muscle so it has a firm, solid feel, it will be easier to find origin and insertion points.

Muscles that usually have the most discomfort include:

HAMSTRING GROUP: Three muscles, located in the back of the upper leg, make up the hamstrings: the biceps femoris, semitendinosus, and semimembranosus. The hamstrings perform certain actions that help with mobility, such as flexing the knee, extending the hip, laterally and medially rotating the hip, and tilting the pelvis posteriorly (toward the back). Common exercises that use the hamstrings are deadlifts, squats, and lower body plyometrics.

QUADRICEPS GROUP: The quadriceps group is one of the more massive muscles in the body. If you look at any bodybuilder, you will notice that this group of muscles tends to be quite large and defined. The quadriceps group consists of four muscles—the rectus femoris, vastus medialis, vastus lateralis, and vastus intermedius, which are mainly used in knee extension. Movements that develop the quadriceps group are leg extensions, lunges, Bulgarian split squats, and power squats.

GASTROCNEMIUS AND SOLEUS: The gastrocnemius and soleus are what make up your calf. The gastrocnemius is the most superficial, while the soleus is deeper than the gastrocnemius. The gastrocnemius has two muscular heads, which gives it a heart-like look when flexed. Located beneath the gastrocnemius, the soleus is an extremely strong muscle because during contraction, it sends blood from the leg to the heart. Most injuries in this area occur at the attachment site, specifically the insertion point, which is the Achilles tendon (calcaneal tendon). If the muscles are too tight, this extremely fibrous tendon junction can tear doing movements like plyometric jumps or even running. The gastrocnemius is responsible for flexing the knee, while the soleus plantar flexes the ankle. Most movements having to do with the quadriceps and hamstrings will inevitably work the gastrocnemius. The most common exercise for development are calf raises.

TRAPEZIUS: Most people associate the trapezius muscles with the two "speed bumps" on either side of the neck. In reality, the triangular trapezius muscles are actually quite large. The origin site is at the occiput—way at back of the neck near the hairline. The unusual part of this muscle group is that the muscle stretches all the way down to the thoracic vertebra, specifically T-12, and this makes up the entire origin site. The trapezius then stretches across to the clavicle and acromion at the spine of the scapula (the top portion), which makes up

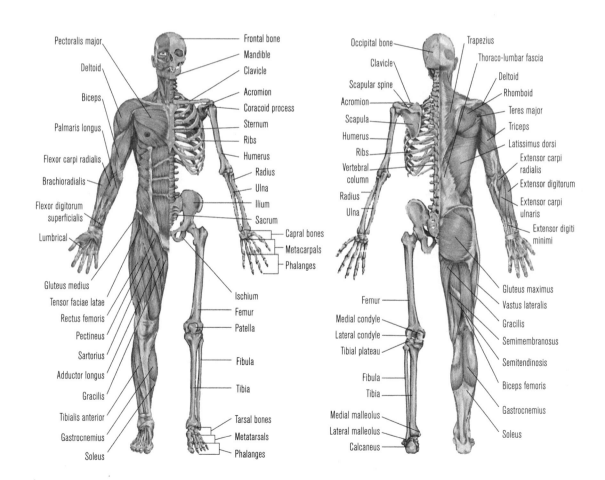

the insertion site. The trapezius is responsible for extending the head and neck, laterally flexing the head and neck toward the same side, rotating the head and neck to the opposing side, elevating the scapula, and upwardly rotating the scapula. There are several exercises that strengthen the trapezius; the most common is shrugs. Banded rows and pull-ups also develop the region.

DELTOIDS: The triangular deltoid makes up the upper shoulder. Deltoids are responsible for abducting the shoulder, flexing the shoulder, medially rotating the shoulder, and horizontally adducting the shoulder. Common movements that strengthen the deltoids are lateral raises, front raises, shoulder presses, and cheerleaders (a front raise to an elbow pull back, then an upward rotation of the shoulder).

BICEPS: Located in the upper arm facing forward from anatomical position, the biceps muscle has a long head and a short head. The biceps have just one insertion site but two different origin sites to accommodate for the two heads. They are responsible for flexing the elbow, supinating the forearm, and flexing the shoulder. The most common movements to strengthen the biceps are biceps curls and concentration curls.

TRICEPS: The triceps are located on the posterior side of the upper arm. The triceps have three heads—long, lateral, and medial. Similar to biceps, the triceps have three separate origin sites to accommodate for the three heads, but only one insertion site. Common movements to strengthen the triceps include lying triceps extensions, triceps kickbacks, and triceps push-ups.

PECTORALIS MUSCLES: The pectoralis muscles make up your chest. There are two muscles in the chest, the superficial pectoralis

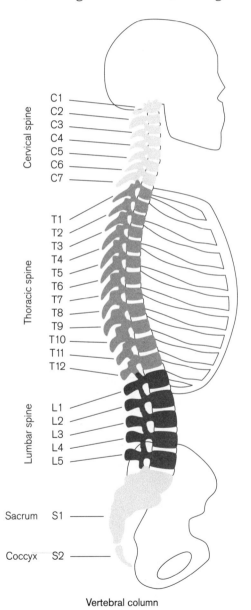

Cervical spine

C1
C2
C3
C4
C5
C6
C7

Thoracic spine

T1
T2
T3
T4
T5
T6
T7
T8
T9
T10
T11
T12

Lumbar spine

L1
L2
L3
L4
L5

Sacrum   S1

Coccyx   S2

Vertebral column

major and the deeper pectoralis minor. The pectoralis major muscle is unique in that the upper fibers and lower fibers perform two different functions. The upper fibers flex the shoulder while the lower fibers extend them. The pectoralis major muscles also medially rotate the shoulder and assist in forced inhalation. The pectoralis minor lies by the rib cage and runs in a perpendicular fashion against the pectoralis major. The pectoralis minor depresses, abducts, and downwardly rotates the scapula, and also assists in forced inhalation. Common exercises that strengthen these muscles are bench presses, push-ups, and dumbbell flys.

RECTUS ABDOMINIS: These muscles are what most people consider the coveted six or eight pack. The rectus abdominis flexes the vertebral column and tilts the pelvis posteriorly. There are many isolation movements to strengthen the rectus abdominis, such as sit-ups, hollow rockers, and knees-to-elbows on a pull-up bar.

Many of these muscles are fairly superficial—meaning they are closer to the surface of the body. Deep muscles, which lie below the superficial muscles, are harder to manipulate.

KINESIOLOGY TERMS

Kinesiology is the study of the human body—specifically, human movement. The origin of a muscle is normally less mobile and is the proximal/medial end of the muscle. The insertion is usually the movable attachment site. In most cases the insertion site is the lateral or distal end of a muscle. For example, the origin of the muscle is usually above (proximal) and the insertion below (distal). You can look at it like this: the origin is a lot like the anchor to the muscle. When you perform a movement, the insertion site aids in the contractile motion of the muscle. Now, this isn't always the case. This is just a rule of thumb when performing a concentric motion. An example of a reversal is a pull-up. The origin of the biceps (scapula) moves up during upward motion, meaning the origin area of the biceps is performing the start of the contractile motion. The radius (insertion of biceps) is the stabilizer of the biceps brachii. In this book, we'll be working with the latter in most cases.

Terms Used in Kinesiology Taping

Become familiar with these terms so that your taping adventure becomes easier.

ANCHOR: This is the start of the taping process. It's applied when the body is in neutral position and has zero tension.

ENDS: This is applied at the end of the taping process. Ends have zero tension.

BASE: This is the area located between the anchor and the end.

TAILS: Anytime tape is segmented into an X, Y, or fan.

INHIBITION: Taping used to relax or elongate a muscle.

FACILITATION: Taping used to shorten or tighten a muscle.

THERAPEUTIC DIRECTION: The direction of recoil toward the anchor.

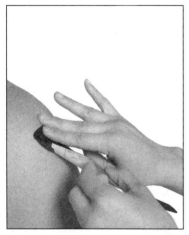 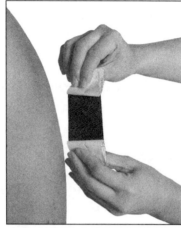 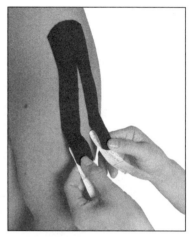

Anchor   Base   Tails

CHAPTER 2
BEFORE YOU BEGIN

The kinesiological tape method serves many uses, but it's primarily used in the stabilization of joints and muscles, to increase the longevity of physical therapy or massage therapy after work has been completed, and for alignment issues. There are several brands of tape that can be purchased, but I find that the Kinesio® brand tape works best for my clients. There are several other tape brands like RockTape, as well as brands you can buy at your local sporting goods stores.

I highly recommend testing out the tape before use because tension strength will differ from brand to brand. Some brands may irritate the skin, depending on a person's skin type, so always do a test run on a small section of skin to see if irritation occurs after one to three days. Always remember, cheaper is not always better in these cases. It's best to buy high-quality tape because it decreases the chances of irritation and usually lasts much longer than generic tape.

There are several different colors of tape that can be purchased depending on the brand. The Kinesio® brand tape uses mainly pink, black, white, and blue. When taping, there's really no difference between tape colors as all have the same wavelike pattern that makes this tape unique to other brands. RockTape has several colors and artistic patterns on the tape—so much so that there are too many to mention here. Other items that could be of use are specific Kinesio® scissors. They're handy to have but not necessary. These scissors are extremely sharp and able to cut through several layers of the Kinesio® tape with precision. They also don't cause the tape to come up from the paper like normal scissors would.

TAPE TENSION

Tape tension can feel a bit complicated at first. I highly recommend cutting a piece of tape and testing out tension. Feel the tape at neutral or zero tension. Then attempt to pull the tape until it's at 100% maximum tension.

Since you'll be using several techniques, attempt pulling tape while one end is anchored; you'll use one hand to actually pull the tape from an anchored position. You'll also attempt to pull the tape with both hands to create "center tension." You'll then adhere the tape with tension in the center. Attempt to create 50% tension at the mid-portion of the tape.

In using this book, you'll be required to judge tension based off of percentages given to you. You may not get it right away but, as you continue to use kinesiology tape, you'll get a better grasp of what the percentages feel like to you. Remember, each brand of tape has a different tension length. I highly recommend that when you find a taping company you like, stick with it. It will help you be consistent in your taping skills.

CLEANING SKIN

Skin must be free of all oils, hair, and lotions before attempting to tape. The tape will not stick if there's any of these on the skin. The easiest way to do this is to purchase basic disinfecting wipes that have no aloe or anything on them. You can also make solutions with a little bit of rubbing alcohol and fragrance-free antibacterial soap.

Clean the area thoroughly. If shaving is needed, you can buy cheaper razors to shave the area (please dispose of them after you have used them—do not reuse razors). Let the skin dry before attempting to tape. If the tape still won't adhere, you can buy what is called "pre-tape" at sporting goods stores. Pre-tape is usually an aerosol canister that sprays a tacky-like substance on the skin to make tape adhere. This is especially beneficial for someone with very oily skin and also aids in the longevity of the tape life on skin. I personally prefer Mueller Tuffner, but everyone will have something they like.

After you've cleaned the area, you can spray a bit of pre-tape and it should be good to go. It's important to mention that pre-tape is extremely tacky and tape will stick extremely well—through rain, showers, and sweat. However, any kinesiology taping should not stay on longer than five days. In most cases, skin irritation will be an unfortunate side effect.

ACTIVATING TAPE

In order to activate the tape, as soon as you complete any taping session, make sure to rub the tape with your hands in order to heat up the tape that you've just completed. Rubbing the tape with your hands warms it up, which in turn activates the acrylic adhesive (depending on which tape you use). I highly recommend that you do this with all tape no matter which brand you use. This also helps with the tape adhering to the body.

CHAPTER 3
BASIC KINESIOLOGY TECHNIQUES

In this chapter, we'll explore the basic taping techniques, or "cuts," used throughout the book. Each project will provide specific instruction on the exact measurements for each taping. This section will break down the basics of mastering each technique.

I STRIP TECHNIQUE

This technique is very easy. The I strip involves cutting the tape the proper length and rounding off the edges. You'll use this technique quite a bit throughout this book. Rounding the edges creates a clean aesthetic, but the round edges can also prevent the tape from catching to other articles of clothing. When people exercise, their sweat can cause the straight edges to start to fray; rounded edges can prevent this from happening.

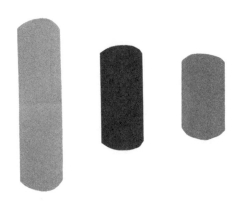

Y STRIP TECHNIQUE

This is a common taping cut you'll use throughout this book and will need to master in order to use some of these techniques. The Y strip is mentioned throughout the book in several ways, including "Y cut." The Y strip technique essentially means you split a piece of tape into two pieces without losing the anchor or base, which remains intact.

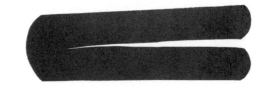

1. Measure your tape to the desired length.

2. Depending on what you're taping, leave roughly 1–4 inches at the end, creating a circular base.

3. Fold the tape in half lengthwise.

4. Use the marking you just made by folding lengthwise and cut the tape in half. Remember to stop at the anchor that you left.

5. Curve the ends that you just created.

FAN CUT TECHNIQUE

Here we'll go over the general idea of lymphatic taping. You can use this taping technique anytime and anywhere on the body that you find swelling or bruising. This is the most basic type of taping that will give you an idea of how tape works, which you'll use when you start doing the most complex techniques. This is a good area to start. You can also purchase pre-made fan cuts online or even in stores.

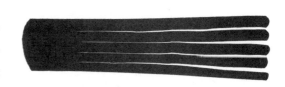

1. Measure the full length of the tape needed for the area of inflammation. Cut tape into five even strips in a horizontal direction until you reach the last 1–2 inches of the bottom of the tape. When completed it will look like a fan.

2. Each area of the body has lymphatic duct draining areas. This is where you'd like the anchor portions of the tape to adhere. Anchor the tape at an area that has healthy lymph traffic on the body, normally proximal to the area of swelling.

3. Apply 0–20% tension on the fan strips on the area of inflammation.

WEB CUT TECHNIQUE

This is another technique you'll use throughout this book. The common mistake with the web cut is cutting through the ends, which is something you don't want to do here. Web cuts are normally used for space-correction techniques in areas of tight fascial structure, areas of pain, and areas with trigger points/adhesions. Essentially, you're creating space in the body where there tends to be tightness due to a variety of reasons. The space correction lifts the skin and thus reduces pressure. Follow these simple steps to create a web cut.

1. Measure out your tape and leave roughly ½–1 inch at the ends of the tape. The easiest way to make sure you don't cut past this area is to use a marker on the paper side of the tape.

2. Fold the tape in half. Cut four strips as evenly as possible. Stop cutting once you reach the stoppage point that you created with your marker. Most kinesiological tapes have grid lines. Use those grid lines to create even strips.

3. Open up your fold to reveal your successful web cut. See page 68 for an example of a web cut.

STAR TECHNIQUE

The star technique is another space-correction technique and used anytime you want to create space as previously described with the web cut technique. This technique tends to use more tension and can be applied anywhere on the body that has pain or where the facia is tight. Large or even small sections of the body, like unsightly scars, can benefit from this technique.

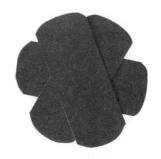

We'll use an example here of someone who has an unsightly scar that they wish to make less noticeable.

1. Create a total of three to four I strips depending on the area that's creating the most pain. Measure out this area and add roughly 2–3 inches to the tape. Some areas may only require three strips; other areas that are increasingly painful may require four.

2. Take one of the strips and break the paper down the center of the tape. Gently peel back the tape so that only the adhesive in the center of the tape is exposed. The paper should remain on the sides. This is important because you're going to use the paper to pull the tape to create tension in the center of the tape. Pulling the tape on the sides with the paper, use 50–75% tension and place the strip directly on top of the scar in the same direction. In this situation, let's say the scar is horizontal. The tails should have zero tension.

3. Take two of the I strips and repeat step two, except now you'll create an "X" on top of the horizontal tape you just used. This will be pretty close to perpendicular to the tape you just placed.

4. This step is optional if the area in question is very painful. Take the fourth strip and place it vertically on top of the X strip and horizontal strip. It should create a "T" pattern with the first tape you placed. Create the same tension as you did in step two.

5. The center of each I strip should overlap with the center of the original horizontal tape from step two. You've created a star, which is a space-correction technique.

DONUT HOLE TECHNIQUE

This fairly new technique is used similarly to the lymphatic technique but has the added benefit of alleviating pain. Its main purpose is to alleviate edema and inflammation. It's important to mention that the actual "hole" in the donut can't be too large. If the center is too large, there's no way to decompress the tissues underneath and thus it can't lift the skin, rendering the technique ineffective.

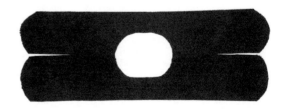

1. After you've measured the area, fold the tape in half. Cut a half circle in the middle of the folded tape. This may take some practice—you don't want too much tape on the sides, but you also don't want too little where it may break. I'd practice with junk tape (tape that may be too short to work with) first.

2. The ends of the tape will be a Y-type cut. You do not want to cut too far into the center or the tape will break. Make a small Y incision and then circle off the ends. Do this to both sides of the tape.

CHAPTER 4
FACE & NECK

In general, the taping techniques offered in this section are for everyday ailments that can occur. Face and neck tapings can be difficult to tape on yourself, so it's best to use a mirror to get your bearings on where tape should be anchored. The only two taping techniques you may need some assistance with are headaches and neck pain. For these particular tapings, I recommend that you release the tape as soon as pain has subsided. Leaving the tape on after that can cause residual effects such as rebound headaches.

HEADACHES

Headaches can range from dull to debilitating. This technique will teach you how to tape for a minor headache, or as a preventative measure for worse headaches and migraines.

Number of tapes: **1**

Shape: **Y strip**

1. Use a Y cut for this type of taping. Leave about an inch at the top and then cut the strip down the middle. First, measure the length of the back of the neck, near the hairline all the way down to the upper shoulders on the medial sides, or toward the upper spine.

2. Now bend the neck forward and look for the occipitus, which is right at the base of the back of the skull. You'll feel it between C1 vertebra and the lower skull, right up the top of the neck near the skull line. Anchor an inch of tape at the upper neck with zero tension.

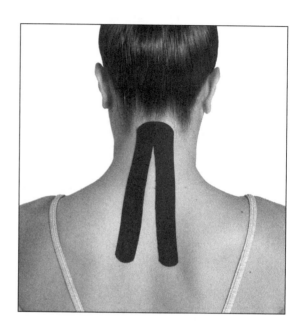

3. Use light tension, around 15–25%, and pull the tails apart on opposite sides of the cervical spine down to the upper thoracic vertebrae. Remember, they should be symmetrical.

4. Spare about an inch of tape at the tail ends (with zero tension at the end).

JAW PAIN

Commonly, pain in the temporomandibular joint (TMJ) region results from grinding your teeth when sleeping or nervously clamping your teeth together. This taping can alleviate some of the pain associated with that. In many cases, people who have TMJ problems will use mouth guards at night to keep them from grinding. Excessive grinding can cause headaches, jaw pain, and broken molars. This technique is fairly easy to complete.

Number of tapes: **1**

Shape: **Y strip**

1. Measure the space between the posterior side of the TMJ, which will be along the jawline near the ear, to about an inch away from the nose.

2. Cut the tape into a Y cut, leaving about half an inch at the top. Anchor the tape at the posterior end of the TMJ.

3. Pull the skin toward the nose, use 10–15% tension on the tape, and pull one part of the Y strip toward the nose and the other along the jaw line. Leave the ends with zero tension.

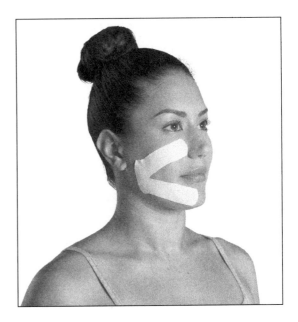

NASAL CONGESTION

Nasal congestion can result from a number of things, including allergies, colds, and the flu. The nasal membranes become inflamed, which can cause blockage or what we experience as a stuffy nose.

> Number of tapes: **2**

> Shape: **I strip**

1. Measure an I strip from the area between the eyebrows to the tip of the nose. Once you measure, fold the tape in half and cut it lengthwise. You'll create, two thinner I strips to use in a smaller area.

2. Place the anchor at the tip of the nose and then peel the tape off using 15–20% tension until you reach the last 1–2 inches. Place the tail between the eyebrow with zero tension.

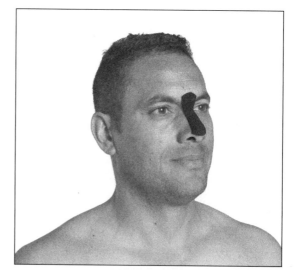

3. Use the second I strip to go across from the right eyebrow arch to the left eyebrow arch. Split the paper of the tape in the center, then gently pull the paper until you reach the tail portion. This will allow you to pull the tape without touching the adhesive. Pull the tape until you reach 15–25% tension at the center of the tape. Release the paper at the two tail ends, using zero tension at the ends.

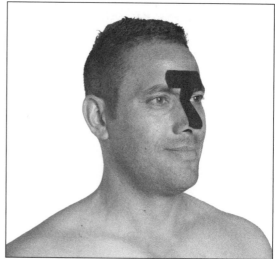

NECK PAIN

This taping technique is for general cervical pain that may be causing headaches, or any neck stiffness that may be due to intense exercise. If you feel that there's serious pain in the area, I recommend that you see your primary care physician immediately.

Number of tapes: **2**

Shape: **I/Y strip**

1. Measure one I strip from the occipitus (the base of the neck) to the upper thoracic spine near the upper shoulder blades. You'll create a Y strip here, leaving about 1" at the top for the base of the neck.

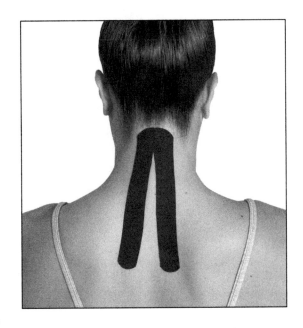

2. Bend the head forward and anchor the Y tails at the mid- to upper thoracic spine on either side of the spine, not directly on it. This area is known as the erector spinae group Once you've anchored both Y strips on either side of the spine, use 15–20% tension until you reach the last 1–2 inches, which should put you at the occipital region. The tail of the tape should have zero tension once you reach this region.

3. Measure an I strip from the bumpy, muscular protrusions on each side of the neck (left upper trapezius to the right upper trapezius). You should measure the tape so that the tape is in the middle of the trapezius before you reach the acromion process (the top of the shoulder). If you reach the bony landmark, you've gone too far.

4. Split the paper on the tape in half (do not split the tape). Once you've split the paper, carefully roll the paper back so that only the adhesive is exposed in the center. Use the paper on both sides of the tape to pull the tape to an approximate tension of 40–70%. Place the tape on the area of discomfort on the neck. The paper will run perpendicular to the tape you put on in steps one and two. Once you have the center of the tape on the area of discomfort, the tails will be left, at which point you'll pull the paper off and adhere the tape on the skin with zero tension.

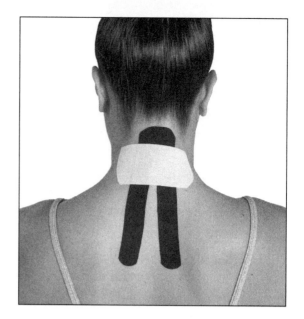

CHAPTER 5
SHOULDER & CHEST

Most athletes or weekend warriors will come into contact with some sort of shoulder pain once in their life. The shoulder typically has issues because of its anatomical design structure. In kinesiological terms, the shoulder joint is a multiaxial ball-and-socket joint, or an enarthrodial joint. It's a joint that moves in all planes. These techniques can be preventative or therapeutic to try with a physical therapist. These tapings can be difficult and may need a second set of hands. As long as you stay seated for these techniques, you can find your way around the shoulder joint.

FROZEN SHOULDER

Frozen shoulder is pain and stiffness in one or both shoulder joints. Symptoms are usually gradual and worsen over time. The risk of frozen shoulder increases if the afflicted individual is recovering from surgery in the shoulder or a specific medical condition. Even though rare, frozen shoulder can develop in the opposite shoulder (remember, the body is bilateral).

This taping technique is a combination taping. You'll be taping more than one muscle.

Number of tapes: **2**

Shape: **Y strip**

1. Prepare two Y strips, leaving about 1–2 inches of headspace. Measure out one tape from the deltoid insertion point to the origin point. (If you flex the deltoid, you'll feel the insertion site close to the middle portion of the arm; the origin site will be close to the top of the shoulder.) Then measure out the coracobrachialis, which is the muscle in the inner portion of the upper arm, up toward the inner portion of the shoulder near the armpit. For the second Y strip, measure from the posterior end of the medial side of the upper, mid-portion of the upper arm (humerus) all the way to the scapula.

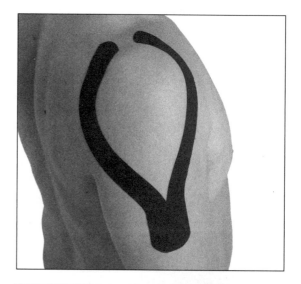

DELTOID—Anchor the tape at the insertion site of the deltoid (deltoid tubercle), which is located at the humerus. Then move the arm away from the body to the side and externally rotate it. Apply 15–25% tension with the Y strips going around both sides of the deltoid. The tails should end up at the medial fibers of the deltoid (posteriorly).

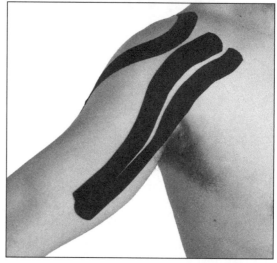

One easy way to find this area is to stop at the top of the shoulder.

CORACOBRACHIALIS—Place the anchor at the insertion site, or medial portion of the humerus in the inner arm. Move the shoulder into abduction and extension. Apply 15–25% tension, moving the tails toward the inner portion of the shoulder near the armpit (coracoid process). You don't want to tape inside of your armpit; you want to trace the shoulder above it. The strips should round the muscle belly and the ends should have zero tension.

ROTATOR CUFF IMPINGEMENT

Rotator cuff impingement is compression of the tendons in and around the shoulder girdle (i.e., biceps tendon and supraspinatus). There could also be a bursa (fluid-filled sac) that applies pressure to the underlying soft tissue and bony structures. If there's inflammation, the soft tissue puts pressure against bony landmarks, causing pain and edema in the area. The main symptom of rotator cuff impingement is pain.

Number of tapes: **2**

Shape: **Y strip**

1. Measure two Y strips. The first you'll measure from the lower deltoid muscle (greater tuberosity of the humerus) to the posterior portion of the trapezius muscles (supraspinous fossa on the medial border of the scapula). You want to stop before you hit your spine. Then you'll measure the same taping as you did for frozen shoulder (page 36).

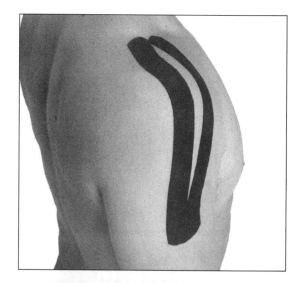

2. Anchor the first Y tape at the lower deltoid. Then move the shoulder into adduction behind the back while flexing the neck in the opposite direction of the shoulder. Apply 15–25% tension on the Y tails, which should both be applied along the medial portion of the scapular near the spine (spinous process of the scapula).

3. The deltoid tape starts out exactly the same as the frozen shoulder taping. This time, the Y tails will go around the shape of the deltoid. The Y tails will end right on top of the shoulder (acromioclavicular joint). You'll feel a bony protrusion in this area.

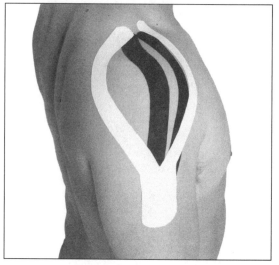

SHOULDER INSTABILITY

This instability usually develops if someone has had his or her shoulder dislocated. It can also happen as a result of overtraining and overuse. This injury can cause a bit of weakness of the tendons and ligaments. Certain exercises can increase the chance of the development of shoulder instability.

Number of tapes: **1**

Shape: **I strip**

1. For this taping technique, you'll use one strip. Measure from the deltoid tubercle, which is at the mid- to upper humerus, to the side of the neck.

2. Anchor the tape at the mid-humerus or deltoid tubercle with zero tension. The tape will remain on the deltoid while the arm is abducted from the body using 35–75% tension on the area.

3. Place the end of the tape near the neck with zero tension and slowly move the arm toward the body.

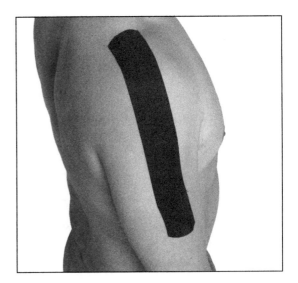

UPPER SHOULDER SPRAIN
(ACROMIOCLAVICULAR JOINT)

You may have heard of an acromioclavicular (AC) joint separation. This ligament injury falls into that particular category and usually occurs when someone falls with their arms open. The symptom of this type of injury is pain at the clavicle. Usually, pain will worsen when you try to use the shoulder in general. Inflammation may occur as well as deformation of the AC joint area. If the pain becomes too great or severe deformation has occurred, always see your physician before using any taping technique.

Number of tapes: **3**

Shape: **Donut hole, I strip**

1. Measure the area of the AC joint, or the top of the shoulder. You'll feel a bony protrusion in this area. You'll use your clavicle and acromion process as reference points. Make the tape slightly longer by just a half inch. You'll create one donut hole taping technique (page 27) for this injury and two I strips.

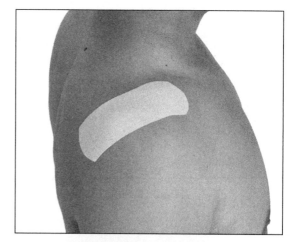

2. Now you'll attempt to make an "X" over the AC joint with the two I strips using 15–25% tension over the area. You're essentially creating the star technique using one strip as a donut hole.

3. The ends of the donut hole tape will be a Y-type cut. Don't cut too far into the center of the tape or it will break. Make a small Y incision and then circle off the ends. Do this to both sides of the tape.

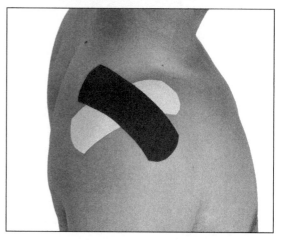

4. After you've measured the area, fold the tape in half. Cut a half circle in the middle of the folded tape. This may take some practice—you don't want too much tape on the sides, but you also don't want too little where it may break. I'd practice with junk tape (tape that may be too short to work with).

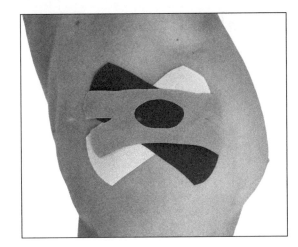

5. After you've completed the donut hole tape, tear the paper portion of the tape in the center. Pull the paper back at the center where the donut hole is and apply 15–25% tension at the center of the tape. The hole part of the tape will be on top of the AC joint going straight through the X you created in step 4 in a vertical fashion. The tails should have zero tension. The Y incision you made will be spread out and not right next to each other. You should create a star on the area.

TIGHT PECTORALIS MAJOR MUSCLE

The pectoralis major muscle can become tight due to muscular dysfunction. How you exercise may cause a "hunchback" look to your body. Common symptoms include trigger points, inability to stretch the chest, and pain in the chest area.

Number of tapes: **2**

Shape: **Y strip**

1. Measure the tape from the lateral edge of the sternum to the front, top portion of the shoulder (humerus near the humeral head).

2. Cut the tape into a Y strip, leaving roughly 2 inches at the end of the tape.

3. Place the hand behind your back to stretch open the pectoral muscles. Anchor one portion of the Y strip at the humeral head and then anchor the second portion of the Y strip right below, about 2 inches down. You'll be taping at the greater tubercle of the humerus.

4. Use 15–25% tension on both strips on the pectoralis major until you have 1–2 inches left and you reach the lateral sternum. The tails should have zero tension.

5. The second part of this taping requires you to measure an I strip from the bottom of the deltoid (deltoid tuberosity) to the top, front portion of the shoulder (acromion process).

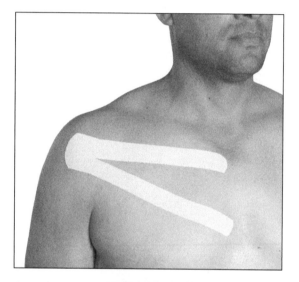

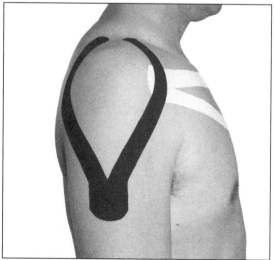

6. Create another Y cut, leaving 2–3 inches at the bottom.

7. Anchor the tape at the deltoid tuberosity. Use 15–25% tension on the first strip, which will cover the front of the shoulder (anterior humeral head), over the initial pectoral tape. Use the same tension on the second strip, which will go on the posterior side of the deltoid. The two tails should meet near the top of the shoulder (acromion process) with zero tension.

CHAPTER 6
BACK & TRUNK

The back and trunk are extremely difficult to tape on your own so I highly recommend that you find a friend to help you with these taping techniques. In regard to anatomy, you can look at the lower trunk as your abdominal muscles, the upper trunk as the chest/rib cage, and the back as your thoracic vertebrae and all muscles attached to it. The vertebral column consists of 24 articulating vertebra and 9 fused vertebrae. The body has 7 cervical discs, 12 thoracic discs, and 5 lumbar discs. The sacrum is a fusion of 5 and 4 fused vertebrae (respectively). (See vertebral column illustration on page 18.)

The trunk is important in that it's a major protection site for organs essential to life. It consists of 12 ribs total that protect all major organs of the upper cavity. We have 7 true ribs as they attach directly on the sternum. We then have 5 false ribs and 2 floating (in general). The manubrium is also part of the trunk in that it consists of the sternum and xiphoid process.

BACK SPRAIN
(Erector Spinae Muscle Strain)

This type of strain is usually caused by poor form during certain movements that are heavy on the low to mid-back. Other causes are high repetitions of a movement that puts a lot of pressure on the low to mid-back. The primary symptom of this is pain and discomfort. Some people may find it difficult to bend over (flex) or overextend the trunk.

Number of tapes: **2**

Shape: **I strip**

1. Measure two I strips that should cover from the sacroiliac (SI) joint to the thoracic vertebrae. The SI joints will feel like two dimples in the back, which are located on either side of the sacrum.

2. You're going to tape on the two sides of the vertebral column. Start by anchoring the tape at the SI joint while in neutral position. Then move into hip flexion and remove the tape at 15–25% tension. The last 2 inches will be the end, which has zero tension. Repeat the technique on the other side of the spine. The two tapes that you put on the back should have a wavelike pattern (convulsions) when the person stands erect.

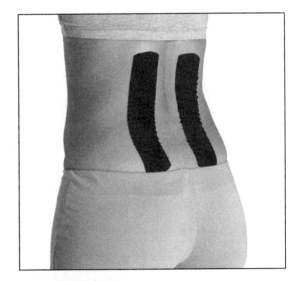

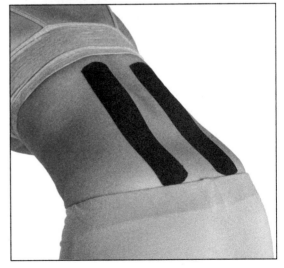

LOWER BACK SACROILIAC PAIN

Pain in this area is fairly pronounced. You'll feel it in your low back near the midline and the medial gluteal region. Certain movements may cause the area to become hypomobile or hypermobile, which can still cause pain during certain movements. Heavy twisting and rotating motions are usually the cause of this. The sacroiliac (SI) joints can become inflamed, which increases pressure on those joints. Pain is felt in the lower back and pelvis.

Number of tapes: **3**

Shape: **I strip**

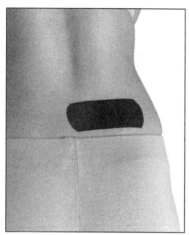 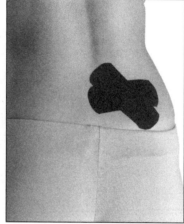 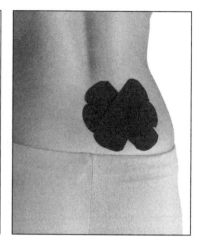

1. For this, you'll apply a space-correction taping. Measure the tape roughly 3–5 inches to cover the sacroiliac joint on your hips.

2. Have the person bow forward (hip flexion). Tear the middle of the tape and use around 25–35% tension on the affected SI joint. (The SI joint will feel almost like a dimple on the low back.) The tails should have zero tension.

3. Measure two smaller, roughly 6-inch I strips and then form an "X" over the SI joint. Tear the tape in the middle with 25–35% tension over the affected joint. The tails will have zero tension. Depending on the pain in the area, you can use more tension, but it isn't recommended to go over 90% on this area.

RIB CAGE SPRAIN
(Costochondral)

A costochondral sprain is essentially a sprain of the rib cage that usually takes place on the lateral sides of the body in the intercostal muscles. Common symptoms are difficulty breathing and pain associated with torsion of the trunk and the thoracic portion of the vertebral column. We'll assume that the inflammation has gone down and is moving toward the post-acute phase. This taping may be difficult to perform on your own so you may need some help from a second party.

Number of tapes: **3**

Shape: **I strip**

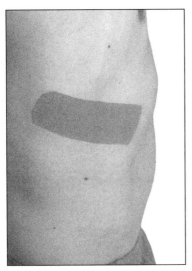 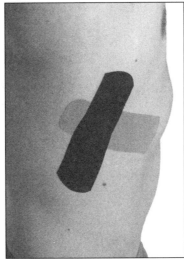 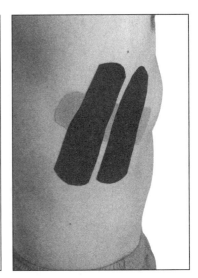

1. You're going to use the I strip technique to tape this area. On the side that's afflicted, move the arm a total of 90 degrees away from the body. The arm should be inline with the shoulder.

2. Measure the tape over the area of pain along the rib cage and tear the tape in the center. The center of the tape will hold the most tension.

3. Place the center of the kinesiological tape over the area of pain with roughly 50–75% tension. Apply the tape at a downward angle, not straight across.

4. Take a full breath, hold slightly, and place the tails on the body without any tension.

5. Cut two more I strips at roughly 6–8 inches and measure the tape so that the I strips will be perpendicular to the previous tape that you put on. One I strip will be closer to the anterior portion of the body, and the second I strip will be on the posterior of the body. Make sure that the I strips are on top of the initial strip without being on the area of tension (the center). Thus, one piece of tape will be visible in the front, the other tape will be visible in the back. Similar to how you taped the ribs, you'll break the paper on the tape at the center, and apply the center of tension on the rib cage. Use 50–75% tension at the center of the tape, take a deep breath, apply the tails with zero tension, and then release.

POSTURAL CORRECTION
(Rectus Abdominis)

This correctional technique is meant to help the person with the tape become aware of their posture and make corrections when their posture begins to waiver. This can be especially useful in events where posture is an important portion of the sport, such as in gymnastics and Olympic lifting.

Number of tapes: **2**

Shape: **I strip**

1. Measure two I strips from the sixth or seventh rib to the iliac crest. You can easily measure both sides of the stomach using the belly button as a reference point. If you have difficulty, you can flex the stomach to see the abdominals protrude a bit and measure the area until you reach the top of the hip bone.

2. Isometrically flex the trunk. You'll facilitate postural contraction by anchoring the tape at the sixth or seventh rib. You'll then tape the rectus abdominis ("six-pack") muscles by taping to the left and right of the belly button. Apply 15–20% tension, leaving roughly 2 inches at the tail with zero tension.

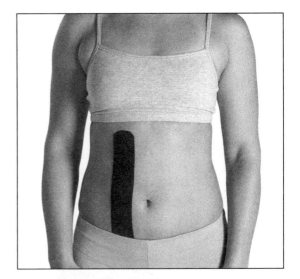

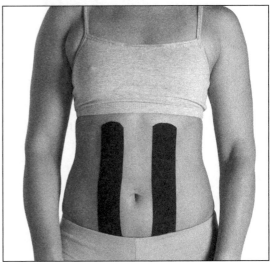

HIP POINTER INJURY

A hip pointer injury is a bruise right on the iliac crest and usually brought upon by direct contact with an object or person. This injury also has some collateral damage, including to the tensor fasciae latae, external oblique, and greater trochanter. Symptomatology includes visible bruising, inflammation, hematoma, and severe pain. If the hematoma and pain become severe, do not tape the area. Please see your physician immediately because the area could have damage to other structures, including deep ones.

Number of tapes: **1**

Shape: **Web cut**

1. Measure an I strip roughly 6–8 inches in length. You'll be taping right over the iliac crest. You can palpate this area by feeling for a hard structure on the top of the hip on the side of the body. When you feel the top of the bony structure, you've touched the iliac crest.

2. You're going to create a web cut. Leave roughly half an inch at both ends of the I strip. Fold the tape in half with the paper side up. Cut the tape in four even strips while leaving the half-inch ends as the stoppage points. Don't cut the tape all the way through the ends.

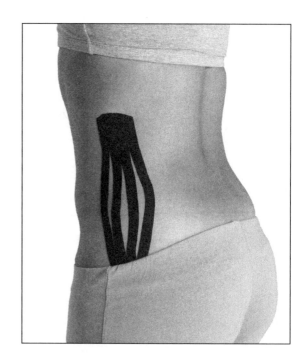

3. Break the paper portion of the tape in the middle where the web cut is located. Place the strips from the web cut on top of the iliac crest using 15–25% tension. Spread the web cut strips only slightly—they shouldn't be far apart. The solid tails should have zero tension at the ends.

MENSTRUAL CRAMPS

This is a bit self-explanatory, but menstrual cramps are also known as dysmenorrhea. The pain can start a week before actual menstruation begins and is usually located in the lower abdomen and lower back. The severity of pain is dependent on the individual. Some have slight pain while others have extreme pain. If the pain is unbearable, renders you immobile, and is complicated by a heavy cycle, please see your gynecologist. This could be a sign of an underlying condition such as endometriosis.

Number of tapes: **3**

Shape: **I strip**

1. First create an I strip roughly 8 inches in length. This I strip will be used for the lower back. Flex the hip by bending forward. Break the I strip paper in the center and gently peel the paper back so that the adhesive in the center is exposed. Use the paper at the ends to pull the tension of the tape to 30–50%. Place the tape at the center of the hip in the lower back. The two tails should reach or surpass the SI joints, which look and feel like two dimples on either side of the lower back near the upper sacrum.

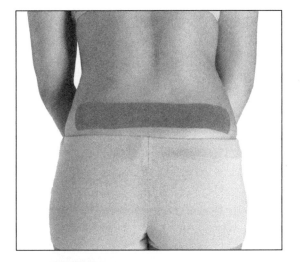

2. Now cut two 6-inch I strips. The easiest way to tape the pelvic region is to lie on your back. Tear the paper in the center as you did in step one. Pull the paper at the ends so you create 20–30% tension at the center of the tape. Place the tensioned I strip horizontally about half an inch below the navel and above the pelvic bone. The tails will have zero tension.

3. For the second 6-inch I strip, tear the paper in the center as you did in step one to

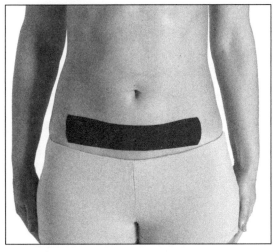

create the tension in the middle of the strip. Create 20–30% tension and place the I strip in a vertical direction on top of the horizontal I strip. Make sure the vertical I strip is in the center of the horizontal I strip. One of the tails should be right below the belly button, and the second I strip should be right near the pelvic bone, both with zero tension. If you accidentally cut the vertical strip too long and the tape goes over the belly button, you can cut the end of the I strip into a Y. Split the Y strip so that the two tails go alongside the belly button.

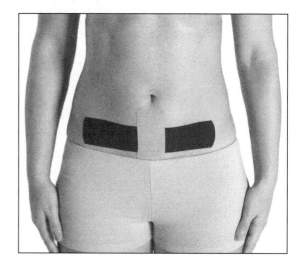

CHAPTER 7
ARMS & HANDS

Arms and hands are fairly easy tapings. You'll be able to tape yourself unassisted. The functional anatomy of the hands is very extensive and we won't be able to cover this information in this book. In general, the human wrist and hand have developed complex mechanisms that allow the hand to move. Roughly, the wrist and hand have 29 bones, 25 joints, and more than 30 muscles (18 of which are intrinsic muscles).

We already know the shoulder is a ball-and-socket joint, but the elbow is different. The elbow is classified as a ginglymus, or a hinge-type joint. The elbow joint only allows for flexion and extension. Since the elbow joint is originally thought of as two interrelated joints, it's also called the radiohumeral joint.

WRIST SPRAIN

As far as structures and function, the wrist and hand are fairly complex . The wrist is classified as a condyloid joint because of its ability to flex, extend, abduct, and adduct. The most common way to get a wrist sprain is by trying to break a fall with your hand. Other ways to get a wrist sprain are through extreme twisting and being hit directly on the wrist. Athletes that usually end up with wrist sprains are basketball players, gymnasts, skiers, skateboarders, snowboarders, and divers. Symptomatology includes swelling, hot to the touch, pain, popping noises around the wrist, and bruising.

| Number of tapes: **3** |
| Shape: **I/Y strip** |

1. Measure a small I strip that will cover the wrist directly on the bony top portion (from the anatomical position, this would be your posterior or extensor side). Measure in the range of 6–8 inches, depending on the person. Tear the paper down the center and gently peel back the paper so that the adhesive is exposed only in the center. The wrist should be at 10 degrees of extension with the fingers separated as far as possible. Use the ends that still have paper to pull the tension to 75–100%. These will be applied on top of the wrist. The tails will go around the wrist with zero tension.

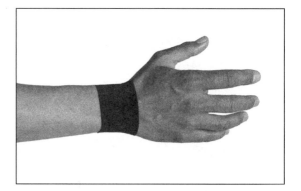

2. Next, measure from the pinky finger (fifth metacarpal) on the wrist area to the medial epicondyle. The medial epicondyle will be in line with the pinky finger on the elbow's medial side from anatomical position. Create a Y cut, leaving 1–2 inches at the bottom. Anchor the solid portion of the tape in line with the pinky finger on the wrist. Fully extend the wrist and use

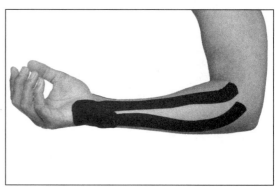

15–25% tension on the Y cut. The two ends of the Y cut should remain fairly close to one another. From the anatomical position, the medial strip should follow the flexor carpi ulnaris, which is just following a straight

line from the pinky finger, and the lateral strip should follow the flexor carpi radialis, which will follow a line near the index finger. Both lines will cross over to reach the medial epicondyle, which is located on a straight line with the pinky finger on the inner elbow.

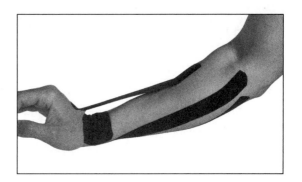

3. Lastly, create another I strip roughly 6 inches long. Fully extend the wrist and anchor the tape at the middle portion of the hand (metacarpals). Do not tape the middle section. This section covers the top of the wrist. Keeping one hand on the anchor, pull the tape so that you create 50–75% tension. Place the tape on the ligament portion of the metacarpals at the tendinous junction of the extensors before you move into muscle tissue. You want to make sure the entire wrist and a little bit of the upper portion of the forearm is not taped over. Leave about 1 inch of tape so that you can put down the tail with zero tension on the meaty portion of the forearm. After you put the tail down, carefully move the wrist into flexion, which should help the tape to adhere to the wrist naturally.

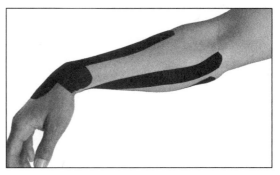

CARPAL TUNNEL SYNDROME

Carpal tunnel syndrome is usually found in those who have jobs that require a lot of typing or usage of the hands. This syndrome involves a pinched nerve in the wrist. Common symptoms are numbness and tingling in the hands and arm. In serious cases, hand and arm weakness can occur and many look toward surgery for treatment. However, there are many treatments offered by physical therapists that can treat the problem without surgical intervention.

You may need the help of another party, but this taping is fairly easy and quick to do.

Number of tapes: **1**

Shape: **I/Y strip**

1. Measure from the thumb and pinky to the lower portion of the upper arm (humerus). You'll want to find the connection of the elbow to the humerus. Cut an I strip and then, about 2 inches down, cut it into Y strips on each end, leaving the I strip in the middle.

2. Tear the center of the I strip. Make sure your arm is completely straight with no bent elbow.

3. After tearing, roll back the tape so that only the center portion is exposed and the ends still have paper on them so you can create tension. The center tension should be roughly 25–35% and in the center of the inner forearm. Keep this tension all the way down to the palm of the hand to all the way up to the elbow, just before the arm bends. The Y cut at the ends will have zero tension, and be sure to split the Y so one side is medial and the other is lateral. The best markers are that one part of the Y

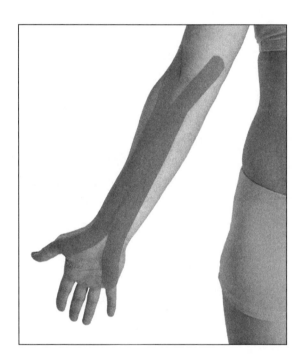

strip is on the pinky and the other is on the thumb. Follow this line all the way up, and the second Y strip will be located along this same straight line along the arm.

LAXITY OF THE ELBOW

Laxity of the elbow is common in those who are hypermobile. Common culprits of laxity of the elbow are repetitive overhead movements, activities that require hyperflexibility, pregnancy, and even sports like baseball or softball. A common symptom is pain. In some severe cases, dislocation is possible. This taping is fairly easy, but you may need the assistance of a second party.

Number of tapes: **1**

Shape: **I strip**

1. Cut an I strip, measuring from the center of the inner elbow and then 4 inches up and 4 inches down.

2. Anchor the tape 4 inches below the upper arm (humerus) and keep your hand on the anchor point. From the anchor, apply about 75–100% tension to the medial elbow (from the anatomical position). For the last 4 inches, use zero tension at the tail.

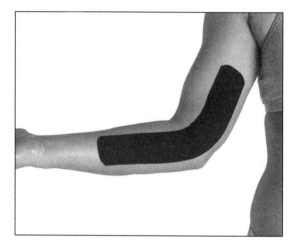

GOLFER'S ELBOW

Golfer's elbow is a condition of the tendons within the elbow region. Symptoms include pain in the inner portion of the elbow, stiffness, weakness, and tingling or numbness.

Number of tapes: **2**

Shape: **Y strip**

1. Measure from the wrist, above the pinky finger (fifth metacarpal), to the inner elbow (medial elbow) when the body is in the anatomical position.

2. Create a Y cut, leaving roughly 2–3 inches at the end of the tape. Anchor this portion of the tape just below the wrist on the medial side at the pinky finger.

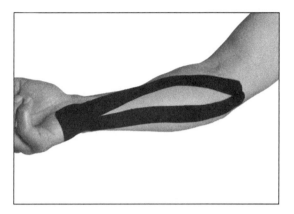

3. Move the elbow into full extension from anatomical position, with the wrist moving slightly back. Use 15–25% tension on both strips. One strip should move toward the ulnar region while the second strip should follow the radial region. (The ulnar region follows the line along the pinky finger, and the radial region follows the line along the thumb.) Both tails should meet at the outer elbow (lateral epicondyle of the humerus).

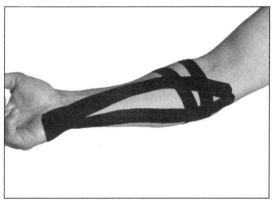

4. The second portion of this taping technique requires measuring another strip roughly 6–8 inches.

5. Create another Y cut, but the I portion will be larger, measuring roughly 3–4 inches. Anchor the I-strip portion of the tape right below the elbow or the area with the most discomfort. Apply 50–75% tension on the I-strip portion. The Y strips will move laterally, spaced fairly far apart, so that the tails are on the inner portion of the arm. The Y strips will have 15–25% tension until you reach the tails, which will have zero tension.

BICIPITAL TENDINOSIS

The biceps brachii are part of two areas: the glenohumeral joint and the elbow joint. The glenohumeral joint is a multiaxial ball-and-socket joint; it's one of the most movable joints of the body. In the glenohumeral joint, the biceps brachii is responsible for flexion and adducting the shoulder in a horizontal direction. The elbow joint is considered a ginglymus joint because of its hinge-type properties. Here, the biceps brachii is responsible for flexing the elbow joint and supination of the forearm. There are two muscles in this group: the long and short head of the biceps. Symptomatology includes pain in the front of the shoulder, weakness, inflammation, and decreased range of motion.

Number of tapes: **1**

Shape: **Y strip**

1. Measure an I strip from below the inner elbow (roughly 1–2 inches) to the area just past the deltoid toward the trapezius. Create a Y cut, leaving roughly 2 inches at the end.

2. Anchor the tape on the area below the inner elbow near the radial head. The easiest way to find the radial head is following a straight line from the thumb all the way up to the elbow. Use 15–25% tension on the Y strips. From the anatomical position, the lateral tape should trace the biceps muscle. The biceps muscle is easy to outline in that you want to move around the muscle that protrudes forward on the arm without taping on top of it. The tail will end up at the top, front portion of the shoulder (supraglenoid tuberosity) with zero tension. The medial side of the Y strip, from the anatomical position, should trace the short head of the biceps without taping on top of it. The tail should end up at the coracoid process, which is toward the front of the

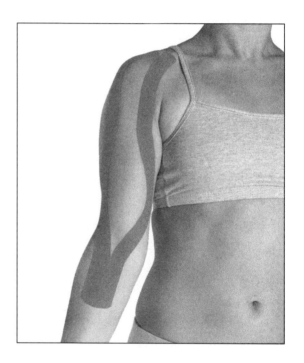

shoulder near the end of the clavicle, in between the front section of the shoulder and the pectoralis muscle. Remember, the tails should have zero tension. When the taping is completed, one tail will be higher than the other, but essentially the tails will be parallel to each other on the shoulder.

BRACHIAL PLEXUS NUMBNESS
(Due to Impingement)

The body has several areas that consist of a plexus, which literally means "braid" and is essentially an area of intermingled nerves. There are more than one plexus and they're located throughout the body. In this case, we'll focus on one in particular. The brachial plexus originates from spinal nerves C5 to T1. Major brachial plexus nerves include the radial, axillary, musculocutaneous, median, and ulnar nerves. Impingement can occur in athletes if they stretch beyond their limit during a collision, experience inflammation, and have tight musculature. Symptomatology includes numbness, tingling, burning, and pain. Be careful with this particular injury. Since you're dealing with nerve pain in this situation, seeing a physician before any sort of treatment may be the best option.

Number of tapes: **1**

Shape: **Web cut**

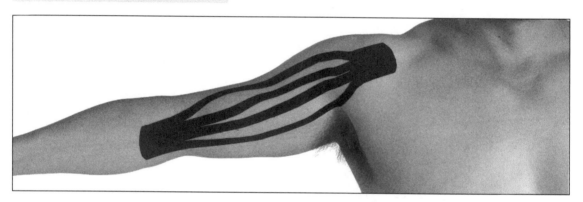

1. Measure an I strip from the inner elbow, right below the crease the elbow makes when bent (aponeurosis of the biceps brachii), to the coracoid process, which is located on the front of the shoulder near the end of the clavicle's lateral side.

2. Create a web cut in order to make a space correction. Leave half an inch on both ends of the tape. Fold the tape in half and cut four even strips. Do not cut the tape like a fan cut—leave the half-inch ends solid so only the middle has the strips.

3. Anchor the tape at the medial side just below the elbow at the bicipital aponeurosis. Make sure the elbow is in full extension. Use 15–25% tension on the web strips. The strips should follow along both the long and short heads of the biceps. The lateral-most strips will trace toward the long head and the medial-most strips will trace toward the short head. Place the tail at the coracoid process with zero tension.

TRICEPS STRAIN

The triceps group has three heads: long, lateral, and medial. Each head has a different origin but the same insertion point. A triceps strain occurs when one of the muscles becomes torn. If the pain is significant and you suspect some sort of rupture, or if the pain does not dissipate over time, please see a health-care professional. Symptomatology includes pain with extension, tenderness to the touch, inflammation, edema, and popping sensations.

> Number of tapes: **2**

> Shape: **I strip**

1. Measure an I strip along the upper arm (humerus) from the elbow to the top of the shoulder. You'll be taping the back of the arm where the triceps group is located.

2. Anchor the I strip at the "funny bone" (olecranon process of the ulna) directly above the elbow. If you hit this area too hard, you may experience a sensation of weakness. Use 15–20% tension as you tape the triceps region until you reach the last 1 inch of the tail near the back (posterior) of the shoulder following the line of the triceps. If this becomes difficult, you can palpate the area to feel the triceps muscle on the upper arm. Stop when you reach the posterior shoulder. Use zero tension on the tape adhering to the skin.

3. Measure another I strip that's roughly 6–10 inches in length, depending on the size of the upper arm. This I strip will be taped in an inside-to-outside (medial-to-lateral) direction. Palpate your triceps muscles to find the area with the most discomfort. Tear the paper of the tape down the middle and

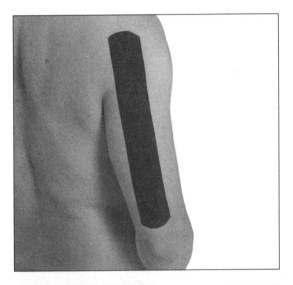

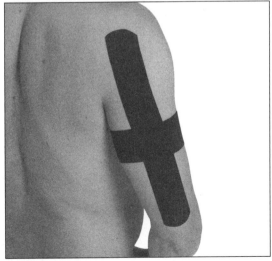

carefully remove the tape, leaving only the ends with the tape still attached. Pull on the paper-covered ends to create 40–60% tension and place them over the area of discomfort. Gently remove the paper off of the ends (tails) and use zero tension to adhere the tape on the skin.

TENNIS ELBOW

Tennis elbow is a condition where inflammation occurs at the tendons of the extensor muscles. Tennis elbow is fairly common in the realm of overuse injuries and is caused by repetitive use of the forearm muscles. Symptomatology includes pain in the outer elbow, pain during stabilization movements, and pain when squeezing different objects.

Number of tapes: **2**

Shape: **Y strip**

1. From the anatomical position, measure the thumb to the elbow on the ulnar side. The ulna traces a straight line from the pinky finger to the elbow. When doing this measurement, you'll cross the inner forearm to the medial elbow.

2. Create a Y cut, leaving roughly 1 inch of an I strip at the end of the tape. Make sure the elbow is in extension before you being taping. The wrist will be bent slightly toward the forearm.

3. Place the anchor at the upper portion of the thumb from the anatomical position. For the Y cut you made, you'll use 15–25% tension. Looking at the thumb, the strip closest to the top of the forearm (extensors) will adhere to that area while the second strip closest to the inner forearm (flexors) will adhere to that area. The tape should be fairly close to each other without being on top of one another. The two tails should meet at the lateral side of the elbow (epicondyle) of the humerus. Use zero tension on the tails.

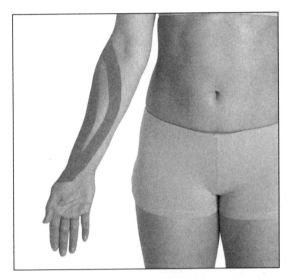

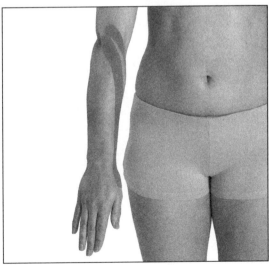

4. The second portion of this taping technique involves measuring an I strip that's roughly 6–8 inches long. Create a Y cut and leave 3 inches of solid strip at the end. Find the area of most discomfort (usually below the elbow) and anchor about 1 inch of the solid portion of the tape right above the elbow. Pull the tape tension at 50–75% only on the solid portion of the tape. Split the Y cut so that the elbow joint is not taped over. Use 15–30% tension on the two Y strips with the tails at zero tension.

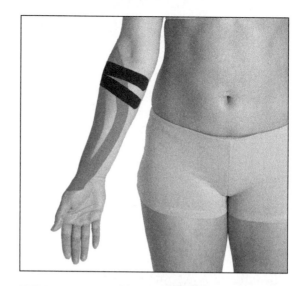

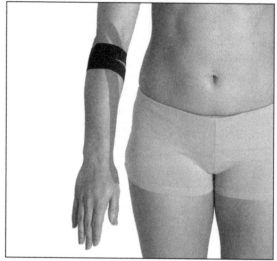

BURSA

Bursas are fluid-filled sacs that manifest in various areas of the body and are quite common in the elbow region. In certain conditions, a bursa can become inflamed; this is called bursitis. In many cases, a bursa will not have any symptoms. The only thing you'll really notice is a raised area that feels like it has fluid in it. When bursas are not attended to, bursitis then occurs, with the most common symptom being pain. In some severe cases, you may find a lack of function in the afflicted area. We'll use two techniques for this: a donut hole and a web cut.

DONUT HOLE

Number of tapes: **1**

1. Measure the tape over the area with a bursa (in this case we'll use the elbow). Bend the arm and measure the tape starting above the elbow and then below it. You'll want 1 inch above the bursa and 1 inch below the bursa.

2. Fold the tape in half. Be sure to round the corners of the ends, and then cut a half circle in the middle of the folded tape. This may take some practice—you don't want too much tape on the sides, but you also don't want too little where it may break.

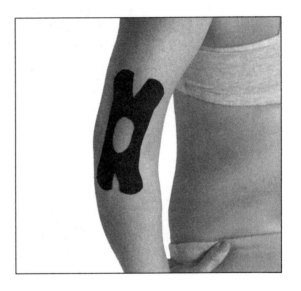

3. Create Y incisions on the ends of the tape. Be careful here—don't cut too far into the tape! You want just a small Y incision, only about half an inch into the tape.

4. After you've completed step three, flex the elbow. Tear the paper portion of the tape in the center. Pull the paper back at the center where the donut hole is and apply 15–25% tension in the center of the tape. The donut hole should be on top of the actual bursa. The tails should have zero tension and will end up on the upper and lower elbow.

WEB CUT

Number of tapes: 1

1. Measure the tape as you did in step one of the donut hole taping. Now cut the tape in half. I highly recommend you cut the tape with the paper exposed—you'll be able to see grid lines that will help you with your cutting.

2. Leave 1 inch at the ends. Use the grid lines to cut four to five slits in the tape for a web cut. Do not cut all the way through. Leave 1 inch on both ends of the tape to use as anchors.

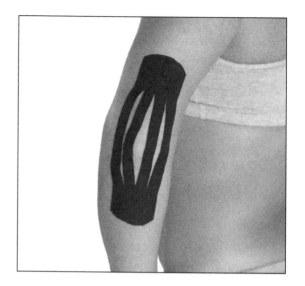

3. Bend your arm and anchor the tape at the top of the elbow. Once you've done this, remove the tape; the web cut should be applied to the bursa area with 10–20% tension. Spread the web cut slightly but not too much to where the web cut is not primarily over the bursa.

4. Anchor the end of the tape at the lower forearm while the arm is still flexed. Since this is the anchor, use zero tension.

Reminder: You can use either the web cut, donut hole, or fan cut technique over any bursa. If you choose a fan cut technique, make sure the anchor portion is above the fan strips toward an area of lymphatic flow or drainage. If the pain is persistent, please see a medical professional.

CHAPTER 8
LEG & BUTTOCKS

The leg area is fairly simple for a single person to tape, but the buttocks may need the help of a second party. Many injuries in this section really belong to the patella in that most people tend to find injury in these places.

The patella is a sesamoid, or floating bone. The quadriceps muscle group, along with the patellar tendon, contains the bone. The knee joint is classified as a ginglymus joint because its function is similar to a hinge (just like your elbow joint). Similar to the elbow, the actual knee joint is called the tibiofemoral joint. The joint itself is made to move between flexion and extension; when it moves beyond these points of action (think very strong side-to-side movements), tears and strains tend to happen. Building strength and flexibility around this joint area can help with stabilization of the knee joint itself.

PATELLAR TENDINITIS

The region of the injury is the tendinous junction of the patellar attachment to the shinbone. You may have heard this injury referred to as jumper's knee, so people that could be at risk are basketball players, volleyball players, long jumpers, triple jumpers, high jumpers, and pole vaulters. Even certain everyday activities like box jumps, wall balls, and burpees can cause patellar tendinitis. For this we'll use a facilitation technique. Facilitation helps weaker muscles by providing support to the afflicted area.

Number of tapes: **1**

Shape: **Y strip**

1. Measure the tape from the origin of the rectus femoris (right below the groin area of the upper leg) to just below the knee.

2. Create an I strip and then split the bottom portion into a Y strip. When measuring, make sure that the knee is bent over an object (like a chair) and cut the Y strip right above the knee to the end of the tape.

3. Anchor the tape at the rectus femoris near the attachment and use 15–35% tension until you get to right above the knee. The rectus femoris attachment site will be a bony protrusion at the lateral-most portion of your hip. If you palpate your hip, you can feel a bony landmark through the skin near the groin area of the body. Tracing this bony protrusion, you'll palpate the anterior inferior iliac spine (AIIS), which is right above the area you just palpated.

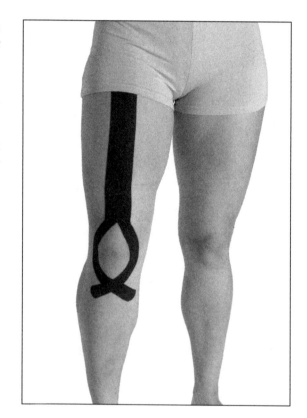

4. Bend the knee deeply, so if you're using a chair, your foot should be at a straight 90 degrees. Your knee should be bent naturally over the chair as if you're sitting with perfect posture. This will make it easier for you to trace the area around the patella as it will be clearly visible.

5. Straighten the leg and apply the tails to the medial and lateral sides of the patella. Cross the extra tails over each other and use zero tension at the tails.

ANTERIOR CRUCIATE LIGAMENT SPRAIN/ DISCOMFORT

The knee joint is classified as a ginglymus joint because it acts like a hinge. The ligaments of the knee provide static stability while contractions of other muscle groups provide dynamic stability. If you're looking directly at the knee, the anterior cruciate ligament (ACL) lies pretty close to the center underneath the patella. ACL injuries are one of the most common and serious injuries to the knee. Studies have shown that these injuries are more common in females than males doing sports such as soccer and basketball. Injuries in this area are from noncontact rotational forces associated with the planting of the lower leg. Symptomatology includes pain, inflammation, inability to walk or bend the knee, and tenderness at the knee. If the pain is severe and walking is impossible, please see a physician immediately.

Number of tapes: **2**

Shape: **I/Y strip**

1. For the first step, you'll use a similar taping technique as for patellar tendinitis (page 70). You'll anchor the tape at the anterior superior iliac spine (ASIS). The ASIS is easy to palpate. When you lie down, you'll feel a bony protrusion near the groin area. It will be more lateral to the body on both sides (remember, our bodies are symmetrical). While the leg is straight, use 15–25% tension until you reach the knee, at which point you'll flex the knee. Split the Y strips using the same tension; one strip will go toward the medial side of the knee without taping on top of the patella. Do the same on the lateral side. The tails should meet below the knee and may cross over with zero tension at the tails.

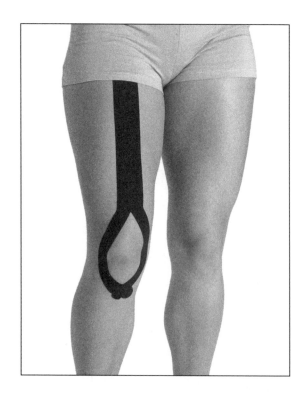

2. For the second portion of this taping technique, create an I strip that measures from the upper, lateral side of the knee to the upper, medial side of the knee. It will be easier to flex the knee to around 30 degrees in order to get a more accurate taping distance. The tape will need to be measured going underneath the knee joint. You'll create a "U" shape, going from the outside to underneath the knee to the medial side.

3. After you've measured your I strip, flex the knee to 30 degrees. Tear the paper down the center and gently peel back the paper so that the adhesive is visible. Use the ends with paper to pull the tape to 50–75% tension. Place the tensioned I strip below the knee at the anterior tibia plateau using downward pressure. The easiest way to remember this area is that it's essentially right below the knee joint. As you begin to put a small section of tape on the knee, begin to bend the knee to 90 degrees as you create a "U" shape that goes around the knee joint itself.

4. Place your hand over the area you taped for leverage. Apply 15–25% tension on the medial side while guiding the tape upward—you're beginning to create the "U" shape. Do the same on the lateral edge until the entire I strip looks like a "U" on the knee. Your "U" shape may not be perfect on the medial and lateral sides, meaning one side of the tape may be longer than the other, but the important part here is creating the "U" shape underneath the knee joint. Use zero tension on the last 1 inch of the tails.

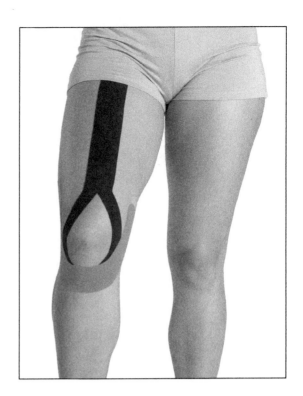

MEDIAL COLLATERAL LIGAMENT SPRAIN

As previously mentioned, the knee joint is a ginglymus joint because of its hinge characteristics. As the name of this ligament suggests, it's located on the medial side of the knee. Sometimes known as the tibial collateral ligament, the MCL is responsible for stability by keeping the knee joint from being abducted. MCL injuries are more common in contact sports such as football, martial arts, and rugby and usually occur when someone falls on the lateral portion of the knee. This causes stress on the medial aspect of the knee in order to keep balance and protection. If this does occur, there could be collateral damage since the MCL is connected to the medial meniscus in its deeper fibers. In regard to symptoms, there are grades in order to assess the damage to the MCL. In this case we'll use grade 1. Usually there's no swelling, but pain, tenderness, and limited movement are common symptoms. Grade 2 and grade 3 require that you see a physician to assess the damage to the area and other collateral damage.

Number of tapes: **2**

Shape: **I strip, 3-strip fan cut**

1. Measure the first strip of tape from the medial portion of the knee near the back of the knee (popliteal region), over the patella, and to the lateral side.

2. You'll be creating something similar to a web cut or lymphatic cut, but you'll be creating three strips lengthwise. Leave roughly 2–3 inches as an I strip and then cut the three strips at an even width. The easiest way to do this is by folding the tape lengthwise into thirds, and then use the folded edges to cut the tape, leaving 2–3 inches at the end.

3. Flex the knee 30 degrees. Anchor the solid portion of the tape at the medial aspect of the knee near the popliteal region

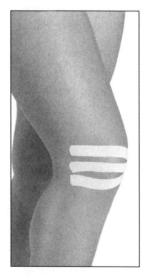
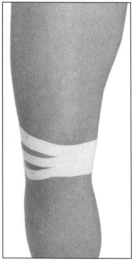

but not on it. While holding the anchor, use 50–75% tension over the inner portion of the knee joint (MCL region). While the knee is still in flexion, the three strips will go over the top, middle, and bottom portion of the knee (using 10–20% tension). The tails will have zero tension on the lateral side.

4. Next, measure an I strip from the lateral, distal portion of the knee (underneath the knee cap) to the inner thighs (upper adductor region).

5. Anchor the I strip on the lateral portion of the bottom of the patella. Flex the knee 30 degrees and use 15–20% tension under the knee. You'll begin to create a "J" shape with the tape you cut.

6. Keep the knee flexed. Hold on to the tape on the bottom of the knee as leverage, and once you reach the MCL (the medial aspect of the knee), use 75–100% tension over the MCL until you pass the medial side of the inner thigh (femoral condyle). You want to stay as close to the medial knee joint as you can. The tape will overlap with the first taping application you used.

7. The third portion of the I strip will only use 15–25% tension up to the inner thighs (middle adductor region). The last 1 inch of the tail should have zero tension.

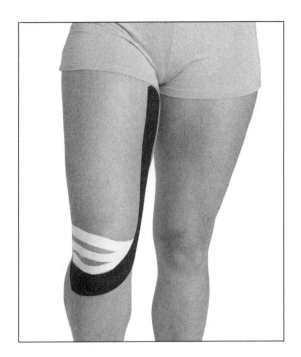

HAMSTRING TIGHTNESS

The hamstrings are located at the back of the leg and are a common injury site for runners, gymnasts, power lifters, and soccer players. When hamstring tightness occurs, it's important to use some sort of preventative action so that no further damage (specifically a hamstring tear) is inflicted on the area.

Number of tapes: **1**

Shape: **3-strip fan cut**

1. Measure an I strip from behind the knee (lower popliteal region) to the ischial tuberosity of the lower gluteal region. The ischial tuberosity will be located in the lower buttocks. This area can be difficult to palpate on yourself depending on body type, but it's the bony section in the gluteal muscles in a downward slope.

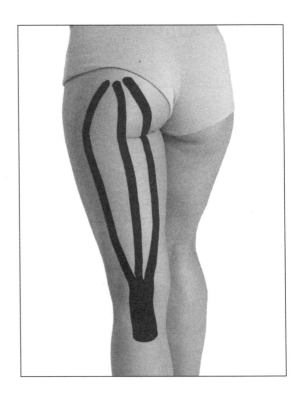

2. You'll be doing a fan cut with three strips. Leave about 1 inch at the bottom of the tape. Fold the tape into thirds and then use the fold lines to create your cuts.

3. Anchor the tape behind the knee (lower popliteal region) near the posterior medial condyle of the tibia. The posterior medial condyle of the tibia will follow a straight line from the big toe to the medial side of the lower leg right before you reach the knee joint. Put the hip into flexion by bending forward at the hip. Use 15–25% tension on each strip. The lateral edge of the strip should trace the lateral side, or semitendinosus. The center strip should stay in the center at the biceps femoris, and the medial strip should follow the medial side, or semimembranosus. You'll trace all three hamstrings with each piece of tape from the cut you created. All three tails should meet at the ischial tuberosity, the protrusions in the lower buttocks region. When completed, the tails should have zero tension.

CHARLEY HORSE

Many athletes and fitness enthusiasts have had a charley horse at least once in their lives. Unfortunately, the cramping is not under our control and can last a few seconds to several minutes. There are a few causes of a charley horse, such as dehydration, not enough minerals, and overuse. The pain can be so severe that some people lose the function of walking when the cramping occurs.

Number of tapes: **2**

Shape: **I/Y strip**

1. Measure one I strip from the heel to the lower portion of the calf muscle (gastrocnemius).

2. You'll then measure a Y strip from the heel to the upper calf.

3. Now stretch the heel flat while the knee is bent. You may need a second party to really stretch the heel or extend the ankle. Apply the I strip with 35–55% tension on top of the Achilles tendon. Anchor the tape with zero tension on the heel of the foot, leaving about 2 inches on the bottom of the foot for the anchor. You want the tape to cover the heel portion of the foot, including the bottom heel.

4. While the knee is still bent and the heel is extended, exposing the Achilles tendon, place the Y strip anchor starting at the heel using zero tension for about an inch. Then add 15–35% tension. Place the two Y strips, one medial and one lateral, around the calf

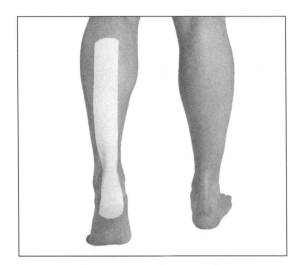

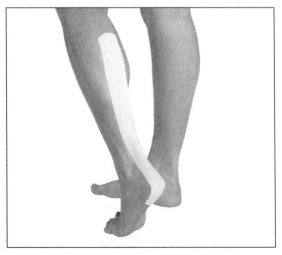

muscle (gastrocnemius). The end tails of the Y strip should have zero tension.

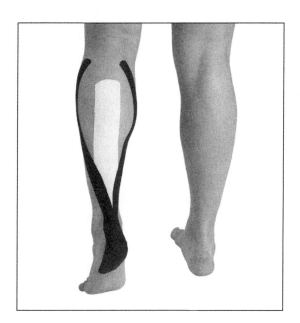

GROIN STRAIN
(Adductor Pain)

A groin strain is due to a sudden forceful action of the muscle or overstretching to the point of tearing. Groin strains are more common in runners, soccer players, football players, hockey players, and Olympic lifters. This injury is mostly uncomfortable and painful. Most individuals feel pain to the touch or while raising the knee and have difficulty bringing both legs together.

Number of tapes: **3**

Shape: **I strip**

1. Measure an I strip the length of the inner thigh, from the groin area to the medial side of the knee joint. There are five different muscles at work during adduction so you want to find the area with the most discomfort. Then measure two more I strips around 6–8 inches in length.

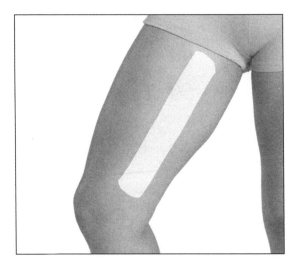

2. To inhibit the adductor muscle, anchor the tape at the medial portion of the tibia with roughly 15–25% tension. Once you reach the last 2–4 inches at the tail, use zero tension in the groin region.

3. Find the area of the adductor muscle with the greatest discomfort. This will be a localized area like a trigger point. Tear the paper of one I strip in the middle. Pull back the paper so the ends still have paper but the middle portion is the exposed adhesive. The tension will be distributed in the middle of the tape—pulling on the ends creates 50–75% tension over the localized area. Gently pull the paper off the ends and use zero tension on the tails.

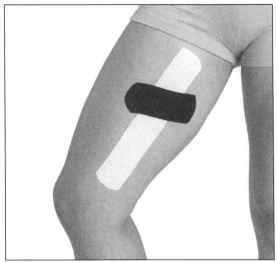

4. Repeat with the second I strip so that your two I strip tapes create an "X" on the area of discomfort in order to create space in the area.

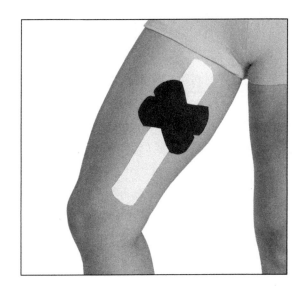

TIGHT ILIOTIBIAL BAND WITH ADHESIONS & TRIGGER POINTS

A tight iliotibial (IT) band (the thick band that runs along the outside of the thigh) can be extremely painful and lead to other injuries. It's quite common in runners, especially endurance athletes. If the area doesn't get properly stretched, the IT band becomes tight, which can lead to IT band syndrome. The symptomatology of a tight IT band includes pain in the knee and/or hip, restless leg, snapping pain over the greater trochanter, and, in serious cases, inflammation.

Number of tapes: **2**

Shape: **I strip**

1. Since the IT band is tight, we'll inhibit the fibrous tissue. Use an I strip and measure the length of the IT band from the anterior iliac crest to the lateral tibia. The anterior iliac crest is located on the side of the body and easy to palpate. It's a hard area on the side of the body that creates a round shape. You'll move your hand forward slightly, which will make it so that the crest is more forward, or anterior, versus posterior. The lateral tibia will be near the lateral side of the knee joint.

2. Anchor the tape at the lateral tibia. Use 15–25% tension over the IT band. Once you reach the anterior iliac crest, the remaining tail will be roughly 2–4 inches long. Use zero tension at the tail to adhere the tape to the body.

3. Palpate your IT band and find the area with the most discomfort. Once you find this area, cut an I strip roughly 6–8 inches

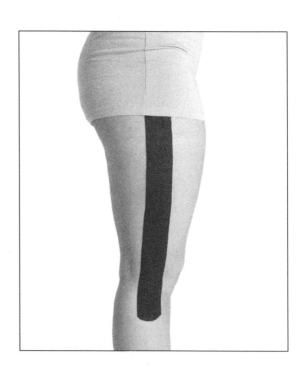

long. You'll be taping in a medial-to-lateral direction with this I strip.

4. Break the paper in the center of the I strip, exposing the adhesive. Carefully pull back the two sections of paper but leave a small amount of paper at the ends to use as your holding points. Pull the tape at both ends until you feel roughly 40–60% tension in the center of the tape. Apply the tensioned tape on the area of discomfort. Carefully pull the paper off the two tails and adhere the tape on the skin with zero tension.

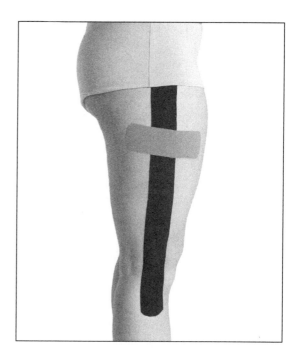

TIGHT PIRIFORMIS

The piriformis is a deep muscle that's a bit narrow and spans from the hip to the sacrum. A tight piriformis is quite common in runners and athletes. Since the piriformis is extremely close to the sciatic nerve (in some cases the sciatic nerve runs right through it), it's important to have a healthy piriformis so that it doesn't cause problems such as sciatica in the future. Symptoms can include numbness down the leg, pain in the buttocks, and overall tightness in the gluteal region.

Number of tapes: **2**

Shape: **I/Y strip**

1. Measure an I strip from the sacrum to the greater trochanter. You can palpate the greater trochanter by finding the upper leg (femur). It will be located on the side of the body, and feel like a round area near the lower hip. Create a Y strip, leaving roughly 1–2 inches at the end.

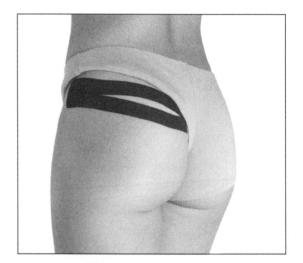

2. Before you begin the taping process, lie down on the side opposite of the leg with the piriformis discomfort. Lift the leg with the knee bent around a pillow to allow the piriformis to stretch.

3. Anchor the tape at the greater trochanter with zero tension. In this technique, the strips of the Y cut will remain fairly close to one another. Use 15–25% tension with one strip on the upper sacrum. The second strip will use the same tension but the tail will be at the lower sacrum near the coccyx (tailbone). The tails will have zero tension.

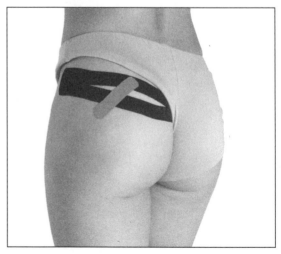

4. Measure one small I strip, roughly 2–4 inches in length. Fold the tape lengthwise and cut the tape in half so that you end up with a thinner taping strip. Find the area of the greatest discomfort in the area you previously taped.

5. Once you find this area, tear the paper on the tape you just created down the middle. Carefully peel back the paper so that the middle potion is the only part that shows the adhesive. Use the paper on the sides to pull tension at roughly 50–75% and put it on the area of discomfort. The tails should still have paper on it, so carefully remove the paper and use zero tension on the tails. If pain persists, you can use an X technique here by taking another thin strip and creating an "X" on the area of the most discomfort.

SCIATICA

The sciatic nerve is the thickest of the nerves inside the body and runs from the lower back all the way down the lower leg so it's no surprise that sciatica can feel very painful from top to bottom. The sciatic nerve eventually splits into the peroneal nerve and the tibial nerve. In most cases, sciatica usually only affects one leg; it's very rare for it to affect both. All people can be effected by sciatica, but it's most common in pregnant women and cyclists. Symptomatology includes numbness or burning from the lower back to the lower leg; some only experience dull pain. It's important to seek medical care if you have difficulty controlling your bowels/bladder while simultaneously experiencing a burning sensation or numbness down the affected leg.

| Number of tapes: **1** |
| Shape: **I strip** |

1. Measure an I strip from the upper gastrocnemius (calf) all the way up to the sacroiliac joint (SI) of the affected leg. The SI joints are small dimples in the low back and can be palpated if you're having difficulty locating this area. You'll want to leave a little extra room in order to tape slightly past the SI joint.

2. Anchor the tape right above the start of the gastrocnemius. Use approximately 1–2 inches as your anchor.

3. Use roughly 15–20% tension as you remove the tape. Keep the tape at the center of the back of the knee (popliteal region) and hamstring group, as the sciatic nerve runs along this line. The tape should run over the center of the buttocks region, or piriformis.

4. Roughly 2 inches of tape should be left as your tail. You'll go over the SI joint and use zero tension in your tail.

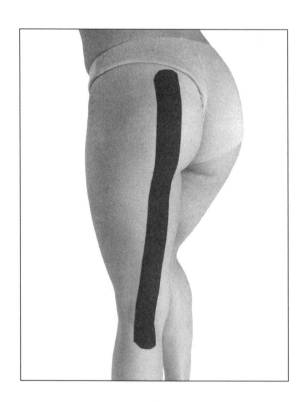

QUADRICEPS CONTUSION

A quadriceps contusion develops when direct and hard contact by another person or object is made with the quadriceps. It's fairly common in contact sports such as football, soccer, and basketball. Broken blood vessels can develop along with crushed muscle tissue. This taping technique is meant to also prevent a very serious condition called myositis ossificans, which is calcium deposits from repeated trauma to a specific area.

Number of tapes: **1**

Shape: **Y strip**

1. Measure an I strip from the anterior superior iliac spine (ASIS) to the area right below the knee. The ASIS is the bony area in the hip near the groin region.

2. Create a Y cut at the bottom portion of the tape. You'll want to have the knee bent so that you can measure this area a bit more accurately. Cut the tape from the bottom until you reach the top of the patella area. The rest of the tape you'll keep as an I strip, as this tape will be covering the quadriceps. You'll be creating a keyhole for this particular taping in that you'll be leaving a bit of tape at the end and not cutting through like a typical Y strip.

3. Use caution for this next part. Anchor the tape below the knee where you created the keyhole cut. Keep the knee bent and anchor the I portion of the tape right below the knee. Using 15–25% tension, use the lateral-most Y cut to adhere to the skin as close to the patella as possible. You'll do the same with the medial side of the Y cut.

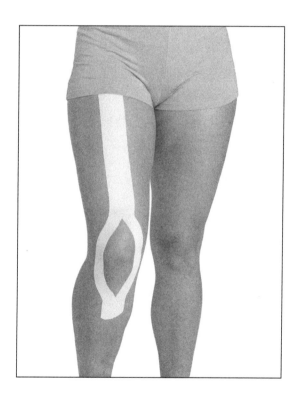

4. Once you reach the I strip portion of the tape, use 15–25% tension all the way up until you have 1–2 inches of tape remaining. Adhere the tail of the tape at the ASIS with zero tension.

KNEE HYPEREXTENSION

Knee hyperextension can be seen in certain sporting events that require flexibility, such as gymnastics, ballet, yoga, and figure skating. For some, knee hyperextension may not be an issue and may even feel natural. For others, mild hyperextension can cause soreness and be slightly uncomfortable. In serious cases, intense knee hyperextension can cause damage to the anterior cruciate ligament (ACL) or posterior cruciate ligament (PCL).

Number of tapes: **1**

Shape: **I strip**

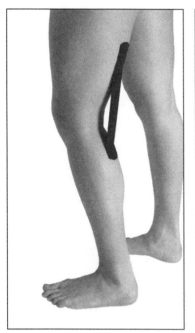 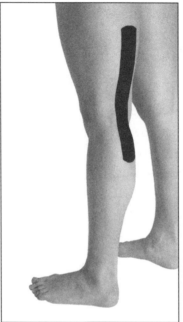 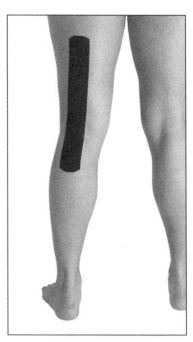

1. Measure an I strip starting at the popliteal region behind the knee. You'll want to measure 4–5 inches of extra tape above and below this region. The tape will hit the femur and gastrocnemius.

2. Flex the knee slightly so that the knee is forward and anchor the I strip at the calf (gastrocnemius) roughly 6 inches below the popliteal region.

3. Apply 30–50% tension and have the tail placed 6 inches above the popliteal region. The tape will not touch the popliteal region yet.

4. While holding both the anchor and the tail, slowly extend the knee so that the tape adheres naturally to the popliteal region. This should help keep the natural anatomical position of the knee.

CHAPTER 9
FOOT

Similar to the hand, the foot is very extensive in structure and too much to cover in this book. The important information is contained here. The foot consists of 26 bones that form the shape of an arch. The bones connect with the tibia and fibula. The human body weight is transferred from the tibia to the talus and calcaneus, where your Achilles tendon is attached. There are five bones known as tarsals that make up the midfoot and the rear. The metatarsals make up the forefoot and the phalanges make up the toes. This may seem like a lot, but each area differs in size.

The ankle joint is made up of the talus, tibia, and fibula. The fibula and tibia form the tibiofibular joint and is classified as a syndesmotic amphiarthrodial joint. You can think of the tibiofibular joint as the area the reaches and attaches to the ankle. The ankle joint in its connection to the foot is called the talocrural joint and is classified as a ginglymus (hinge) joint. It only allows for flexion and extension at limited degrees, so many injuries tend to happen when there's a diversion to the function of the joint (for example, pivoting and landing in an unnatural position).

These taping techniques can alleviate pain from these accidents and help restore stability by placing the joint in the correct anatomical position. If the injury is too severe, you need to see a medical doctor immediately.

ACHILLES TENDINITIS

Anytime you see "-itis" at the end of the word, it usually means some sort of inflammation. In this case, we're talking about inflammation of the Achilles tendon. This overuse injury is most common in runners, ultrarunners, and triathletes. Luckily, this type of injury very seldom requires medical attention and can easily be treated at home.

Number of tapes: **1**

Shape: **Fan cut**

1. Measure an I strip from the heel of the foot to the lower hamstring. For this taping technique, you'll want to leave 2–4 inches from the start of the soleus to the foot for the bottom measurement.

2. Measure from the lower heel (calcaneus) down to the end of the tape. Perform a fan cut in this area of the tape. Use the backside of the tape to see grid lines. Use those grid lines to make four strips at the end of the tape.

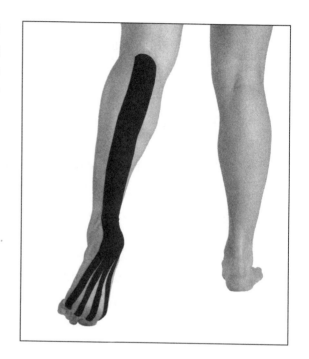

3. Make sure the foot is dorsiflexed. Tear the tape at calcaneus, near the fan strips you just created. Place the tape at the heel with zero tension. The fan cuts will adhere to the bottom of the foot while you place 75–100% tension to each fan cut. Spread the tape out so that each fan cut is near each toe, but on the padded area of the forefoot. Leave the end of the tails and anchor them with zero tension.

4. To tape the ankle and calf, use 50–75% tension on the Achilles tendon in a straight line while leaving 1 inch at the top. Use the last bit of tape as an anchor with zero tension.

PLANTAR FASCIITIS

Plantar fasciitis is the inflammation of the fascia on the bottom of the foot. It can be debilitating and feel like you're walking on broken glass. Most people feel the most pain in the morning when the fascia tends to be tightest. By afternoon, some of the pain usually dissipates because the fascia has had a chance to warm up and become more pliable. This is not the case for all who have plantar fasciitis, though. Some have pain no matter what time of day it is.

Number of tapes: **2**

Shape: **Y/I strip**

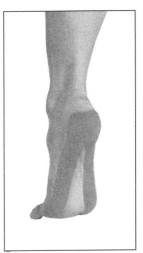
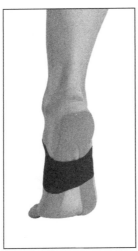
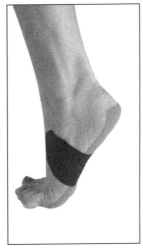
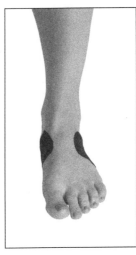

1. Measure from the heel of the foot to the padded portion of the forefoot. You'll leave the heel with a solid strip, roughly 2 inches. Cut a Y strip that leads down to the forefoot.

2. Anchor the tape at the heel. Using roughly 15–25% tension, split the Y cut so that one strip follows the line of the pinky toe and one follows the line of the big toe. You don't want the tape to adhere to the toes; you want the tails to reach the padded portion of the forefoot. Once you reach this area, use zero tension to put the tails down on the foot.

3. Measure an I strip that wraps around the bottom of the foot to the top of the foot without the tape overlapping. Find the place on the foot with the most discomfort. Break the paper portion of the tape in the middle. Using 25–75% tension, use the base of the tape on the bottom of the foot. Wrap around the tape so that the tails have zero tension on the top of the foot.

BUNION

A bunion is found on the medial edge of the big toe right at the base where the joint is located. It forms when your big toe pushes against the toe next to it, creating a protrusion at the joint of the big toe. Quite common in ballet dancers, gymnasts, and skaters, bunions can be painful, especially if the incorrect shoes are worn. When a bunion forms, it's important to wear shoes that are wider at the toe box. Symptomatology includes pain, swelling, redness, corns, calluses, and restricted movement.

Number of tapes: **2**

Shape: **I/Y strip**

1. Measure an I strip the length of the medial side of the big toe to the back of the lower Achilles heel (calcaneal tendon).

2. Anchor the tape at the big toe with zero tension. Apply 15–20% tension on the I strip until you reach the large protrusion on the side of the ankle (malleolus). Here, the tail will adhere to the calcaneal tendon with zero tension.

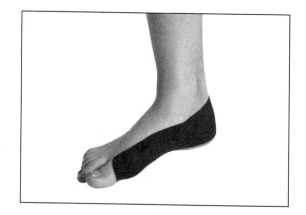

3. Next, measure an I strip that goes from the bunion to the pinky toe. You'll then cut the tape in the form of a Y strip, but leave a significant portion—about 6 inches—as an I strip. The I strip portion will adhere to the top of the foot.

4. The Y strip should split in two: the top strip around the top potion of the bunion and the bottom strip around the bottom portion of the bunion. The strips should be relatively close to the bunion without being directly on top of it. Use 20–35% tension on the Y strips, leaving roughly 1–2-inch tails

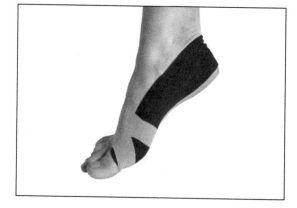

with zero tension. The I portion of the strip will cover the top of the foot at the metatarsophalangeal joints. Use the same tension strength here as well, leaving the tail with zero tension.

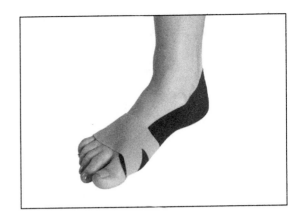

LATERAL ANKLE SPRAIN

The most common of ankle sprains, lateral ankle sprains are damage to the ligaments on the outer edge of the ankle. These sprains are popular among soccer players, basketball players, volleyball players, and runners. The most common symptoms are pain and swelling. There are three different grades when it comes to ankle sprains. In this case, we'll use grade 1. Symptomatology includes mild pain, some instability, light joint stiffness, and slight difficulty with walking/ running. If you feel you have a grade-3 sprain (a complete tear of the ligament and zero stability in the joint), see your physician immediately.

If swelling has occurred, you can use the lymphatic taping technique (page 25) first before taping for post-acute injuries.

Number of tapes: **1**

Shape: **I strip**

1. While in dorsiflexion, measure from the bony protrusion on the medial side of the ankle (malleolus), under the arch of the foot, to the lateral side right below the knee. This will be an I strip technique so round the ends.

2. On the lateral edge of the knee, begin with an anchor that uses zero tension. After you've anchored your tape, begin to use 15–35% tension. Follow the tibialis anterior as a guide as you move the tape down toward the foot.

3. This part may be slightly tricky. Plantar flex the foot while at the same time moving the foot into eversion. You'll still use 15–35% tension as you go over the lateral malleolus to the bottom of the foot. Make sure the tape goes on at the arch of the foot.

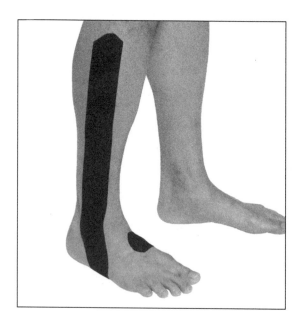

4. As the tape goes around, you should have the tape meet at the medial malleolus. From there, anchor the tape with zero tension.

MEDIAL ANKLE SPRAIN

Medial ankle sprains are fairly rare, occurring when the ligaments and tendon of the medial portion of the ankle are stretched or torn. This injury normally occurs in those who run "pigeon-toed," or with the feet everted. Symptomatology includes pain, swelling, difficulty with weight bearing, bruising, and little range of motion.

Similar to lateral ankle sprains (page 94), during the acute phase you can use lymphatic taping (page 25) to help reduce swelling.

Number of tapes: **2**

Shape: **I strip**

1. You'll use an I strip technique with this. Measure from the lateral mid-portion of the side of the foot (around the area of pinky toe) and then go under the foot to about a half inch past the bony protrusion on the medial side of the ankle (malleolus). Make sure the foot is in a relaxed state.

2. With the foot in a neutral or dorsiflexed position, anchor the tape at the lateral blade of the pinky toe using zero tension.

3. Use 15–50% tension while going along the arch portion of the bottom of the foot to the medial malleolus. Once you meet the medial malleolus, use zero tension and anchor.

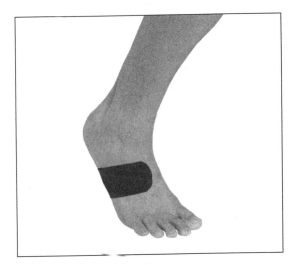

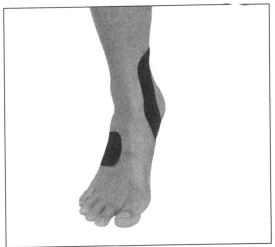

4. Measure a second I strip from the lateral malleolus, underneath the arch of the foot, all the way up to the medial portion of the knee. Start the tape around the lateral malleolus then dorisflex and evert the foot. Using 15–35% tension, guide the tape to go underneath the foot from the lateral malleolus to the medial knee. Anchor the tail with zero tension.

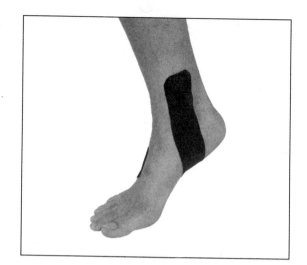

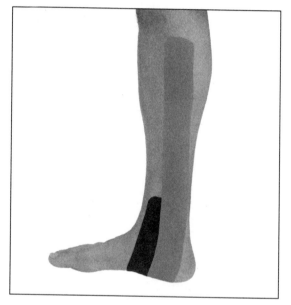

RESOURCES

Mueller Tuffner Pre-Tape
www.muellersportsmed.com

Kinesio® Tape Pre-Cut Strips
www.fab-ent.com

Kinesio® Tex Tape
kinesiotaping.com/www.shopkinesio.com

Clinical Therapeutic Applications of the Kinesio Taping Method by Dr. Kenzo Kase, Jim Wallis, and Tsuyoshi Kase

Kinesio Taping Perfect Manual by Kinesio Taping Association

PowerTaping: Theories and Practical Applications of Fascial Movement Taping by Dr. Steven Capobianco and Greg van den Dries

Kinesiology Taping: The Essential Step-by-Step Guide by John Langendoen and Karin Sertel

BIBLIOGRAPHY

Biel, Andrew. *Trail Guide to the Body,* 3rd edition. (Boulder, CO: Books of Discovery, 2005), 29–224.

Capobianco, Steven, and Greg van den Dries. *PowerTaping: Theories and Practical Applications of Fascial Movement Taping.* (Los Gatos, CA: RockTape, Inc., 2013), 42–79.

Floyd, R. T. *Manual of Structural Kinesiology.* (New York: McGraw Hill Companies, 2012), 1–20, 118–201.

Kenzo, Kase, Jim Wallis, and Kase Tsuyoshi. *Clinical Therapeutic Applications of the Kinesio Taping Method,* 3rd edition. (Albuquerque, NM: Kinesio, 2013), 13–270.

Kenzo, Kase, Jim Wallis, and Kase Tsuyoshi. *Clinical Therapeutic Applications of the Kinesio Taping Method,* 2nd edition. (Kinesio Taping Associates, 2003), 201–203.

Kenzo, Kase, Hashimoto, Tatsuyuki, and Okane, Tomoki. *Kinesio Taping Perfect Manual: Amazing Taping Therapy to Eliminate Pain and Muscle Disorders.* (Kinesio Taping Associates, 1996), 106–107.

Tate, Philip. *Seely's Principles of Anatomy and Physiology.* (New York: McGraw Hill Companies, 2012), 310–320.

Werner, Ruth. *A Massage Therapist's Guide to Pathology,* 3rd edition. (Baltimore: Lippincott, Williams & Wilkins, 2005), 648–650.

INDEX

ACKNOWLEDGMENTS

I'd like to thank my family for all the support they have shown me throughout the writing of this book. Thank you Pete Pfannerstill, PhD, LMT, CKTI, for teaching me the Kinesio Taping® Method this book is based on. I'd also like to thank the Kinesio Taping Association International—this book would not exist without their support and expertise. Thank you Claire, Casie, and the entire staff at Ulysses Press for making this dream a reality.

ABOUT THE AUTHOR

Aliana Kim has worked in health care and rehabilitation most of her adult life. She studied biology at the University of North Carolina and then began her higher level education in kinesiology at the University of Nevada at Las Vegas. In her free time, Aliana enjoys reading, exercise, hiking, and spending time with her husband and two dogs, Marley and Tanner.